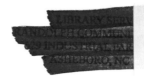

D0859864

Preterm Babies, Fetal Patients, and Childbearing Choices

Basic Bioethics
Arthur Caplan, editor

A complete list of the books in the Basic Bioethics series appears at the back of this book.

Preterm Babies, Fetal Patients, and Childbearing Choices

John D. Lantos and Diane S. Lauderdale

The MIT Press
Cambridge, Massachusetts
London, England

25.65

MIT Press books may be purchased at special quantity discounts for business or sales promotional use. For information, please e-mail special_sales@mitpress.mit.edu.

This book was set in Stone by the MIT Press. Printed and bound in the United States of America.

Library of Congress Cataloging-in-Publication Data

Lantos, John D., author.
Preterm babies, fetal patients, and childbearing choices / John D. Lantos and Diane S. Lauderdale.
    p. cm. — (Basic bioethics)
Includes bibliographical references and index.
ISBN 978-0-262-02959-9 (hardcover : alk. paper)
I. Lauderdale, Diane S., 1955– , author. II. Title. III. Series: Basic bio-ethics.[DNLM: 1. Premature Birth—etiology—United States. 2. Infant Mortality—trends—United States. 3. Infant, Premature—United States. 4.Obstetrics—trends—United States. 5. Prenatal Care—United States. 6. Reproductive Behavior—United States. WQ 330]
RJ250
618.3'97—dc23
                                                                2015009281

10 9 8 7 6 5 4 3 2 1

618.397
Lan

Contents

Series Foreword

Glenn McGee and I developed the Basic Bioethics series and collaborated as series coeditors from 1998 to 2008. In Fall 2008 and Spring 2009 the series was reconstituted, with a new Editorial Board, under my sole editorship. I am pleased to present the forty-sixth book in the series.

The Basic Bioethics series makes innovative works in bioethics available to a broad audience and introduces seminal scholarly manuscripts, state-of-the-art reference works, and textbooks. Topics engaged include the philosophy of medicine, advancing genetics and biotechnology, end-of-life care, health and social policy, and the empirical study of biomedical life. Interdisciplinary work is encouraged.

Arthur Caplan

Acknowledgments

This book has had a decade-long gestation. It would not have been possible without a grant from the Robert Wood Johnson Health Policy Investigators Program. That grant would not have been possible without discussions about the problem of preterm birth that we had with many colleagues at the University of Chicago. William Meadow and Larry Casalino made valuable comments on our earliest proposals to study the problem of preterm birth. The RWJ program not only provided funding for the project but also provided an opportunity to present our work in progress at annual meetings to a group of attentive, critical, and helpful scholars.

We were lucky to work with Tyler VanderWeele and Juned Siddique. Both helped design and carry out the empirical analyses about changes in childbearing over the last few decades that formed the first stage of our project. Both were lead authors of papers whose results informed our evolving understanding of preterm birth. Scott Moses gave valuable feedback on an earlier draft of the manuscript. Katharine Lauderdale created the figures for the book.

We were given opportunities to try out the arguments in the book at medical conferences and grand rounds presentations at the University of Chicago, Children's Mercy Hospital in Kansas City, Northwestern University, Vanderbilt, and meetings of the American College of Epidemiology and the Pediatric Academic Societies.

1   Two Narratives about Pregnancy in the Twentieth Century

A little girl is born weeks before her due date. Her mother looks at the new tiny person and worries about her future. She is such a fragile little wisp. Will the prematurity cause problems down the road? Will her eyes or her lungs be weak? Will she have trouble in school? Will she have emotional problems? Her mother worries about when her baby will be able to leave the hospital. She is afraid that breast-feeding will be impossible.

In addition to all these worries about the baby, the new mother also has another set of worries. She wonders whether her baby's early arrival was her fault. Was there something about her own health and her actions during pregnancy that caused this? Was it the flu she had in the fifth month? The acetaminophen she took for headaches before she knew she was pregnant? She has been stressed at work and having trouble sleeping. Could that have caused the premature birth? Was all this preventable?

She is also grateful. She is grateful for the technologically sophisticated obstetric care that enabled her to see ultrasound images of her tiny fetus. On the ultrasound screen, she could see the heart beating. She could count the fingers. She could sort of see that her baby looked normal. She was grateful for the technology that monitored the infant during delivery. She knew that, but for the miracle of modern neonatal intensive care, her baby would probably not have survived. Preterm infants like hers all used to die. Now they can grow strong and go home, cooing and crying like normal, full-term babies. Now they can go on to live happy, normal lives.

While her baby is in the neonatal intensive care unit (NICU), a mother's every day is a rollercoaster of emotions. In any single hour, she will feel fear, guilt, gratitude, anxiety, hope, and confusion. She will be told things that are reassuring and things that she doesn't understand. She will be addressed with sensitivity and with condescension. She will sometimes feel supported. At other times, she will feel judged. She will absolutely love some of the nurses. Others will always be just "the blond one" or "the mean one."

Many parents in the United States go through such experiences after a premature birth. The United States has one of the highest rates of premature birth among industrialized nations. Our preterm birth rate is nearly twice as high as in many European countries (though preterm birth rates are rising in Europe, too).[1] The percentage of babies born preterm in the United States (11.5%) is closer to the rates found in India (12.9%) or Ethiopia (10.1%) than the rates found in France (6.7%) or Sweden (5.9%).[2] Within the United States, rates vary greatly by race and ethnicity. In 2012, the preterm rate was 10.3% for non-Hispanic white infants and a similar 10.2% for Asian and Pacific Islander infants, but 16.5% for non-Hispanic Black, 13.3% for American Indian and Alaskan Native and 11.7% for Hispanic infants. Note that *all* of these rates are higher than European rates.[3]

Although the preterm birth rate in the United States has stopped increasing in the past five years, and has even ticked downward, it remains much higher than in comparably wealthy countries. In 2012 the state with the lowest preterm birth rate, Vermont, still had a higher rate than almost every European country. Even with the recent decline, the preterm birth rate could be seen as one of the major public health failures of the United States in our time.

This book is an exploration of why so many preterm babies are born in the United States, why the rate has risen over the last few decades, and why, even though preterm birth is a leading cause of infant mortality, the U.S. infant mortality rate has been steadily falling. We have two central theses. One is that the problem of premature birth is complex and multifactorial. It cannot be understood as simply a medical problem or a social problem or a problem of access to prenatal care. There are no simple solutions and no single solutions to prevent preterm birth. Some of the immediate causes of early birth can be attributed to the mother and her health and health behavior. Other causes reflect larger contextual factors that have contributed to our very high rate of preterm births, factors that include social and cultural changes. They also include changes in the clinical practices and the technologies used in obstetrics and pediatrics. We will even suggest that some of the most widely touted and ardently defended responses to the problem of premature birth, such as increased emphasis on comprehensive prenatal care, may paradoxically lead to more premature births rather than fewer.

That leads to our second thesis in the book. Premature birth may not mean what it meant a few decades ago. Then, reducing preterm birth was a priority because it was a means to reducing infant mortality. The correlation between premature birth and infant mortality today is not as tight or as straightforward as it used to be. As the preterm birth rate rose in the United States over the last few decades, the infant mortality rate fell. This can be seen in figures 1.1 and 1.2. The first graph shows that infant mortality rates dropped from 6.91 in 1,000 in the year 2,000 to 6.05 per 1,000 in 2011, a 12% decline.[4]

The second graph shows that during those same years the preterm birth rate reached an all-time high. Between 1981 and 2008 it rose nearly 20%, from 10.5% to 12.6%.[5] Over the last five years, the preterm birth rate has started to drop. Neither the early rise nor the most recent fall seems to have had much effect on infant mortality.

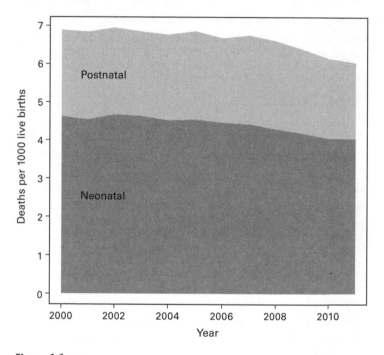

Figure 1.1
Neonatal and postnatal mortality rates in the United States, 2000–2011. Source of data: Martin JA et al., Births: Final data for 2012. National vital statistics reports; vol 62 no 9.

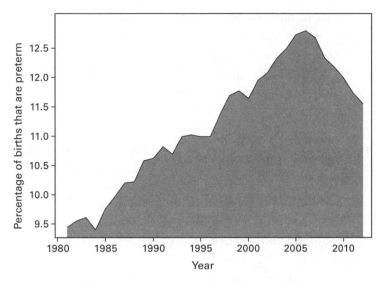

Figure 1.2
The U.S. preterm birth rate from 1981 to 2012, showing an increase from 1981 through 2006 and then a steady decline since 2006. Source of data: Martin JA et al., Births: Final data for 2012. National vital statistics reports; vol 62 no 9.

For at least thirty years, then, we have had rises and falls in the rate of preterm birth accompanied by steadily falling rates of infant mortality. We will examine the implications of these trends in preterm birth rates and infant mortality in detail and try to figure out why our preterm birth rate remains high and why, in spite of that, our infant mortality rate is getting steadily lower.

One factor that may be crucial is that over the last half-century there have been many changes in the ways that we go about having babies in the United States. Women have fewer babies over the course of their lives than they used to. As demographers

would put it, our total fertility rate is falling. Women are having babies at a different stage of life. More women are delaying
childbearing than ever before, so the average age of women at
the time of childbirth is going up. There are fewer births to teen-
age mothers today than at any time in our history. More people
use effective contraception, so the number of pregnancies and
the number of births for the average woman in the United States
is lower than ever. These changes have been made technologically possible by better techniques to control fertility. Advances
in prenatal diagnosis and the legalization of abortion have made
delayed childbirth possible without the otherwise inevitable rise
in the number of babies born with chromosomal anomalies. We
will explore the impact these changes have had on the rate of
preterm birth.

Our exploration leads to a surprising realization. Preterm
birth, while obviously not desirable, may no longer be synonymous with a bad birth outcome. Rates of preterm birth have
long been a focus of attention because they served as a surrogate measure for tracking the much lower infant mortality rate,
allowing researchers and policy makers to identify trends, and
differences between population groups, that could not be seen
as clearly from an examination of infant mortality. Preterm birth
was considered a key preventable cause of infant mortality, even
though prevention has not been very successful. If the trends in
preterm birth and infant mortality do not move in parallel, then
it is less clear what preterm birth rates tell us. The fact that the
rate of preterm birth has risen while the rate of infant mortality
has fallen shows, at the very least, that preterm birth is not a
measure of the risk of infant mortality on a population level. The
corollary is that preventing preterm birth may not necessarily
bring about a lower rate of infant mortality.

Another interesting feature of childbearing in the United States today, one that is less widely publicized than the preterm birth rate or the infant mortality rate, is that the rate of fetal mortality—that is, of stillbirth—has also fallen dramatically over the last thirty years. Fewer pregnancies end in stillbirth today. This change, which we discuss in more detail in chapter 3, has enormous implications both for individual decisions and for public health policy.

Our analyses raise questions about some of the conventional wisdom about pregnancy, childbirth, and infant mortality. To focus these questions, we suggest that two very different and competing narratives have been told about the development of the modern American way of pregnancy and childbirth. These narratives are at odds with one another.

One is the story of women's long march to reproductive freedom. This story begins with Margaret Sanger's rejection of her mother's Catholicism, her civil disobedience, and her brave attempts to provide birth control to all women who wanted it. It goes on to tell how Sanger collaborated with scientists and philanthropists to develop the oral contraceptive pill. The story then shifts from the laboratory to the courtroom, where litigators eventually convinced the United States Supreme Court to strike down laws that prohibited women from buying birth control, which led to the eventual legalization of abortion and the establishment of women's right and ability to control their own fertility and their own bodies. The same values allow women today to choose to schedule their cesarean deliveries, to have their babies in hot tubs, or to avail themselves of in vitro fertilization. By this story, these are the best of times. Pregnancy is safer than ever for women, and infant mortality is lower than it has ever been.

A counternarrative sees modern obstetrics as fundamentally hostile to women. By this telling, women are the victims of a culture in obstetrics that has turned pregnancy into an illness. The empowering phenomenon of childbirth has been transformed into a disempowering experience in which unnecessary medical interventions are provided in settings that prohibit women from having their babies in a healthy way. This view of pregnancy and childbirth today sees the rising rate of C-sections and medical inductions of labor as a sign of the abject failure of the entire enterprise, one that harms women and leads to outcomes for both women and babies that are far worse than in other industrialized countries.

Tellers of the first story point to the dramatic drops in pregnancy-related mortality and in complications of delivery such as incontinence, sexual dysfunction, and chronic abdominal pain. Tellers of the second story point to the fact that maternal mortality rates have leveled off or perhaps even begun to rise in the United States and are higher than in most European countries.

In these debates about obstetrics, the focus is typically on women. In this book, we will try to connect changes in reproductive health care, contraception, and obstetrics with outcomes for babies. In particular, we will examine infant mortality rates and preterm birth rates in order to see whether changes in obstetrics are making things better or worse for babies. Here, too, different stories can be told. On the positive side, the infant mortality rate in the United States is lower than it has ever been. More than 99 of every 100 live-born babies now live to see their first birthday. On the negative side, our infant mortality rate in the United States remains much higher than in many other countries. More problematically, racial disparities in survival rates, always large, are getting bigger rather than smaller.

This book is an attempt to make sense of these competing stories by analyzing the facts that lie behind them. It began as an attempt to understand why prenatal care did not seem to be working the way it was supposed to work. Better access to prenatal care was supposed to lead to lower rates of preterm birth. But more women get prenatal care today, and they get more of it than ever. What went wrong?

Preterm birth has long been recognized as the leading cause of infant mortality and morbidity. Preterm babies who survive are at heightened risk for a lifetime of medical problems and medical costs. Both preterm birth rates and infant mortality rates are among a small number of markers or "sentinel events" that are used to measure the overall efficacy of a nation's health care and social welfare systems. For many policy analysts, measuring preterm birth rates is like taking the temperature of a nation. The implications of high rates of preterm birth go beyond purely medical considerations. Higher national rates of preterm birth or infant mortality can be correlated with many other national characteristics and indexes (though not necessarily in a cause-and-effect relationship). Countries that spend a higher percentage of their GDP on their militaries have higher rates of infant mortality.[6] Better access to clean water and effective sewage disposal are associated with lower rates of infant mortality.[7] Countries with more teachers in their schools have lower rates of infant mortality. These sorts of associations do not necessarily reflect causation or, if they do, it may be direct or indirect. But the associations are suggestive of the symbolic ways in which high infant mortality rates are seen as a sign of a sick health care system—or a sick society. Lower rates signify that the health care system and, by analogy, the society that creates and supports it, is working.

The World Health Organization publishes international rankings of preterm birth rates that look like the standings of sports teams in a league. By these rankings, the United States should have fired our coach long ago. We have been falling slowly and steadily in the international rankings for the last thirty years. The frequency of preterm births is now about 12% in the United States and 5% to 9% in most other developed countries.[8] The comparison can be seen in figure 1.3.

Preterm birth is defined as birth before 37 weeks of gestation, measured from the woman's last menstrual period. Low birthweight—that is, birthweight of less than 2,500 grams—is not synonymous with preterm birth, although the terms are sometimes used as if they are interchangeable. A baby can be preterm but weigh more than 2,500 grams, or low birthweight but full term. However, there is significant overlap between the two classifications. From a public health perspective, either can be used to monitor health policies, although a third category, "small for gestational age" is also used to describe low birthweight, full-term infants. Preterm birth rates are generally higher than rates of low birthweight because many babies born close to term have "normal" birthweight. Even when preterm birth is the conceptually preferred metric, low birthweight may be used because weight is almost always accurate on birth records while gestational age may be imprecise.

Our failure to reduce the rate of preterm birth has not been for lack of effort. Like a drumbeat, national commissions periodically recognize and highlight preterm birth as a significant medical and public health problem. Those reports invariably set ambitious goals of reducing preterm birth or low birthweight. Often, they recommend concrete mechanisms for achieving that goal.

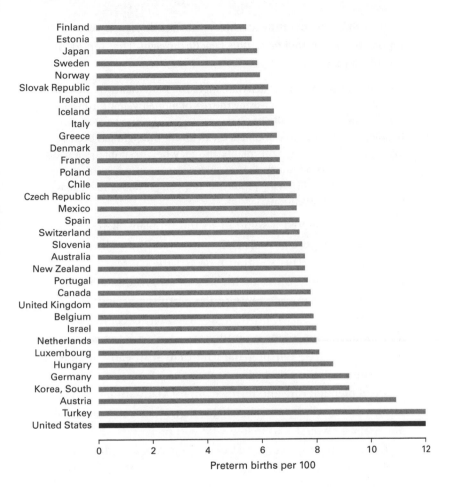

Figure 1.3
Preterm birth rates in 2010 among countries in the Organisation for Economic Cooperation and Development (OECD). Data based on Liu L, Johnson H, Cousens S, et al., Global, regional, and national causes of child mortality: an updated systematic analysis for 2010 with time trends since 2000. *Lancet* 2012;379:2151–2161.

In 1985, the Institute of Medicine (IOM) issued one such report. It was entitled *Preventing Low Birthweight.* That report laid out the stark facts,

Low birthweight is a major determinant of infant mortality in the United States. In addition to increasing the risk of mortality, low birthweight also increases the risk of illness...The association of neurodevelopmental handicaps and congenital anomalies with low birthweight has been well established; low birthweight infants also may be susceptible to a wide range of other conditions, such as lower respiratory tract infections, learning disorders, behavior problems, and complications of neonatal intensive care interventions.[9]

The report offered a solution to the problem. Better access to prenatal care, the authors claimed, would lead to lower rates of preterm birth. This solution reflected the consensus among experts at the time who saw the lack of access to prenatal care as the major correctable cause of low birthweight and preterm birth. Epidemiologists noted that "low birthweight, neonatal mortality, and infant mortality were 1.5 to 5 times greater with late, less frequent prenatal care than with early, frequent care. Multivariate analysis demonstrated a positive relationship between prenatal care and birthweight."[10] Many studies showed similar associations and echoed the claim that better access to prenatal care would lead to lower rates of preterm birth.[11]

The IOM report argued that expanding Medicaid to provide better access to prenatal care would not only be effective in reducing low birth weight and preterm birth but would also be cost-effective. The authors argued for the following causal chain: (1) poor people without health insurance were less likely to seek and receive prenatal care than wealthier, insured people; (2) programs to provide insurance to poor people would lead to higher rates of prenatal care; (3) higher rates of prenatal care would lead to lower rates of preterm birth; (4) lower rates of preterm birth would mean less need for expensive neonatal intensive care, which was already paid for by government insurance programs; therefore, (5) increased access to prenatal care would lead to a net cost savings for government insurance programs. The IOM estimated that every dollar spent on prenatal care would save $3.37 in neonatal care expenses. This led one legislator to conclude, "It is not often that a person in public life gets to say, 'I know how to save the lives of American children and save taxpayer money at the same time.'"[12]

In response to this report, Congress passed legislation in the late 1980s providing funding to expand the Medicaid program in order to improve poor women's access to prenatal care.[13] This legislation passed with bipartisan support. President George H. W. Bush signed it into law.

In one sense, the Medicaid expansions worked. More poor women did, in fact, enroll in Medicaid, and more of these women received prenatal care. From 1990 to 2003, the percentage of women who received prenatal care during the first trimester of pregnancy increased in all racial and ethnic groups. Over these years, the percentage of pregnant women who received no prenatal care was cut in half.[14]

But in a more important sense, these Medicaid expansions did not work at all. National rates of both preterm birth and low birthweight birth continued to rise during the same years.

In 1991, the U.S. surgeon general issued a report, "Healthy People 2000," setting ten-year goals for the nation's health. One of the goals was to reduce the rate of low birthweight births from 6.9% to 5%. Over the ensuing decade, the rate rose to from 6.9% to 7.6%.[15] Undaunted, the surgeon general issued a new set of goals, "Healthy People 2010," calling once again for a reduction in low birthweight to 5%. That report also called for a reduction in preterm birth from 11.6% to 7.6%. Over the next years, both low birthweight and preterm birth continued to rise. In 2007, the IOM issued its own report. Once again, the authors presented the compelling case for a new national effort to reduce the rate of preterm birth. They noted,

Infants born preterm are at greater risk than infants born at term for mortality and a variety of health and developmental problems. Complications include acute respiratory, gastrointestinal, immunologic, central nervous system, hearing, and vision problems, as well as longer-term motor, cognitive, visual, hearing, behavioral, social-emotional, health, and growth problems. The birth of a preterm infant can also bring considerable emotional and economic costs to families and have implications for public-sector services, such as health insurance, educational, and other social support systems. The annual societal economic burden associated with preterm birth in the United States was at least $26.2 billion in 2005.[16]

In 2008, in a third report, the Surgeon General of the United States echoed the IOM's call for more attention and research to the problem of preterm birth.[17]

And the preterm birth rate continued to rise.

Over these years, the relative international ranking of the U.S. infant mortality rate steadily worsened.[18] In 1960, only a few European countries had lower infant mortality rates than the United States. Now, we are not in the lowest fifty.[19] We seem to be even worse at perinatal health care than we are at soccer and math.

Preterm birth is one of the leading causes of infant mortality. So it seemed that our failure to prevent preterm birth was one of the reasons why we were also unable to lower our rate of infant mortality. By 2010, CNN could report that

The United States has the second worst newborn mortality rate in the developed world, according to a new report. American babies are three times more likely to die in their first month as children born in Japan, and newborn mortality is 2.5 times higher in the United States than in Finland, Iceland or Norway. Only Latvia, with six deaths per 1,000 live births, has a higher death rate for newborns than the United States, which is tied near the bottom of industrialized nations with Hungary, Malta, Poland and Slovakia with five deaths per 1,000 births.[20]

What has gone wrong? Better access to comprehensive prenatal care for more pregnant women was thought to be the best means to reduce the rate of preterm birth and thus the rate of infant mortality. But improved access to prenatal care did not seem to be helping in the way it was supposed to help. The United States kept trying harder but seemed to be moving in the wrong direction.

In order to investigate what was behind this phenomenon, we sought and were awarded a grant by the Robert Wood Johnson Foundation's Health Policy Investigator Program. Our project was entitled "Prenatal Care: Wise or Wasteful?" We set out to examine whether prenatal care was an ineffective waste of money. Our inquiry began as a narrowly focused analysis of the content and the efficacy of prenatal care. It gradually expanded. Prenatal care, it turns out, has changed dramatically over the last 100 years. There are many reasons for that. Some reflect advances in technology such as amniocentesis, fetal ultrasound, or intrauterine fetal monitoring. Others reflect changes in patterns of childbearing, particularly the tendency of women today to delay childbearing until they are older. That tendency leads to both infertility and higher-risk pregnancies.

We realized that preterm births had also changed. Many preterm births now are medically induced. We needed to explore the ways that obstetricians think about the risk of stillbirth and the benefits of induced preterm birth. Those risks cannot be understood without also analyzing the rise of neonatal intensive care. So the problems of prenatal care, preterm birth, and infant mortality must be understood in the context of a long and complex story about the ways that we go about having babies and how that has changed in the past century.

Our inquiry into the causes of preterm birth grew broader. During the last decades of the twentieth century, people were changing the way they thought about and organized family life. Marriage did not mean what it used to mean. Career paths were different. The demographic makeup of our society was changing. Many of those changes were related to the rising rates of preterm birth—some as cause and some as effect. It was hard to make sense of the story of rising preterm births without placing it in the context of a society in which so many other things were changing. So the two narratives of childbearing do not tell the whole story. Instead, it is a story with a number of subplots, many possible protagonists, and ambiguous heroes, heroines, and villains.

One subplot began in 1913, when the newly formed Children's Bureau of the Department of Labor issued its first handbook on prenatal care. That handbook expressed a clear view of the role of prenatal care. After extensive discussions of diet, exercise, and psychological health, the book concluded, "If the pregnant woman lives in such a manner as to establish and conserve her own health, taking plenty of sleep and exercise, eating sensibly of simple food, and in every way striving to take the best possible care of her own body so that the digestive, assimilative, and excretory functions are carried on in the highest degree of efficiency, she can be quite sure that the child will be able thereby to build up for himself a sound and normal body and brain."[21] This was the prevailing view of prenatal care through-out most of the twentieth century. It is the view that informed the 1985 IOM report. Prenatal care was seen essentially as a preventive sort of therapy focused on the health and well-being of the pregnant woman.

Another subplot began a few years later, in 1916, when Margaret Sanger was arrested for daring to dispense birth control in a clinic she had started for that purpose in New York City. Sanger also wanted to improve the health of babies and mothers. She sought to do so by giving women some control over their fertility so that they could limit the number of babies they bore and thus bear healthier ones. Forty-four years later, scientific research inspired by Sanger led to the first FDA-approved oral contraceptive pill.

An important chapter of the story we tell about the ways that we go about having babies concerns the events of 1942. In that year, Wilson demonstrated that supplemental oxygen could improve respiratory status in premature babies.[22] This breakthrough marked the beginning of modern neonatal intensive care. The development of neonatal intensive care would eventually lead to therapies that would reduce infant mortality not by preventing preterm births but by saving preterm babies who were dying of respiratory distress syndrome and other problems associated with prematurity. The next big advance in the neonatal care piece of the story came in 1964, when Delivoria-Papadopolous and colleagues in Toronto showed that they could intubate the trachea of a dying premature baby and keep her alive using intermittent positive-pressure ventilation.

Other highlights of the narrative include the work of Jerome Lejeune and that of Arthur Liley. In 1959, Lejeune showed that Down syndrome was caused by an extra chromosome, a discovery that led to amniocentesis and the ability to diagnose a variety of diseases in the fetus. Liley developed techniques to measure bilirubin levels in amniotic fluid and to perform intrauterine blood transfusions on babies with Rh disease. With these extraordinary interventions, for the first time the fetus became a patient, whose treatment was separate from that given to the pregnant woman.

Liley's work to make the fetus a patient who could be treated was given a further nudge in 1962 when Hon showed that he could continuously monitor fetal heart rate patterns. He began to understand the relationship between fetal heart rate abnormalities, fetal distress, and stillbirth.[23] Nadler's 1968 report of the first diagnosis of trisomy 21, made using cultured cells from amniotic fluid, was a key development in the evolution of prenatal care from a purely preventive treatment to one focused on diagnosis of diseases in the fetus.

These discoveries had complex ramifications. They expanded the range of choices available to women. Safe, effective, and available birth control allowed women to control their fertility. The ability to diagnose fetal disease and fetal anomalies allowed women not just to manage their fertility but also, to a certain extent, to have healthier babies; or, conversely, to know when the health of a fetus was so impaired that it made sense to terminate the pregnancy. The ability to diagnose fetal disease in these new ways allowed obstetricians to tell pregnant women if their babies would be born with severe congenital anomalies. This knowledge was a key component of the rationale and cultural support for the legalization of abortion.

A new chapter in the long story of changing reproductive practices began in 1970 when the Boston Women's Health Collective published the first edition of *Our Bodies, Ourselves*. That book would change the ways that women thought about pregnancy and childbirth. It encouraged women to discuss health and sexuality with each other, to learn about the medical controversies associated with common practices in obstetrics and gynecology, and to question some of those practices.

All of these developments form the story of changes in the ways in which we have babies. Direct assessments of fetal health and wellbeing allow obstetricians to make decisions based upon those assessments, and to calculate the benefits and risks of particular interventions for the fetal problems they have diagnosed. Sometimes, these assessments lead to the conclusion that the best thing to do for both mother and baby is to medically induce a preterm delivery. The net effect of these changes has been to sever the previously tight connection between preterm birth and infant mortality. Today, those two measures no longer move in lockstep. Even as preterm birth rates have climbed steadily higher, infant mortality rates have just as steadily dropped.

These changes are interconnected. A woman's decision about when to bear children used to be heavily influenced by the relationship between advancing maternal age and higher risk of chromosomal anomalies, especially Down syndrome. The discovery of the chromosomal cause of Down syndrome, the invention of techniques to diagnose it in early pregnancy, and the subsequent legalization of abortion made it possible for women to think about having babies in their late thirties or early forties without increased risk of having a baby with a chromosomal anomaly.

Such developments have had some unanticipated consequences. Women who delay childbirth are more likely to have problems with fertility than younger women. Infertility treatments such as medications that stimulate ovulation or the use of in vitro fertilization (IVF), developed in the 1970s and 1980s, allow childbearing at older ages. These drugs also increase the rate of multiple births and preterm births. Furthermore, women who are in their thirties or forties when they have babies are at higher risk of delivering preterm than are women in their twenties, even without IVF or twin pregnancies.

Advances in prenatal diagnosis and in the treatment of infertility led to new questions about the moral status of the fetus. The better we get at seeing the fetus, and at diagnosing and treating fetal diseases, the harder it is to make absolute moral distinctions between the fetus and the newborn. We end up with the paradoxical formulation that the fetus can be a *patient* without being a *person*. Arguments ricochet back and forth between the clinic and the courtroom about the implications of diagnosing and treating newborns with congenital anomalies or babies born at the borderline of viability. Should such babies be treated even though treatment is very expensive and outcomes are not always good? Should parents, or doctors, be permitted to let such babies die? How and why do moral obligations and legal restrictions change at the moment of birth? What is the legal or moral significance of that moment of marvelous transition from intrauterine to extrauterine life? Many of the doctors who pioneered the interventions that allow us to diagnose fetal disease were, or became, profoundly opposed to abortion.

Different ways of telling the stories of these developments lead to different conclusions about the implications of our rising rates of preterm and low birthweight birth. They suggest different solutions. Our understanding of the problems and our decisions about how to respond are shaped by the fact that all the debates surround very personal decisions and choices by millions of women and men about sex, love, babies, and families. Thus, discussions of law and policy, though inevitably political, are also deeply personal. Technical discussions of the science of reproduction eventually lead to new options that shape the world of anyone who wants to have a baby. Many of the key players in these stories have taken an intensely personal interest in the outcomes. So this book became a story not only about science and health policy, but also of individuals and their struggles.

Specific developments occurred against the backdrop of the dramatic scientific and societal changes that took place during the second half of the twentieth century. Many of those changes, indirectly but profoundly, changed the way we think about health and disease, reproductive choices, infant mortality, and public health.

In 1953, Watson and Crick discovered the structure of DNA, or, in Crick's words, "the secret of life."[24] The next year saw the introduction of the polio vaccine. At that time, contraception was still illegal for unmarried women in most states. (Of course, it was only technically illegal. Since the late 1930s, birth control had been widely available, even through federally subsidized programs.[25])

The year John F. Kennedy was elected president was also the year the FDA approved the first birth control pill. By 1968 some colleges were dispensing birth control pills through their student health services. That year, Pope Paul VI addressed his "venerable brothers ... and all men of good will" with these words: "The most serious duty of transmitting human life, for which married persons are the free and responsible collaborators of God the Creator, has always been a source of great joys to them, even if sometimes accompanied by not a few difficulties and by distress."[26]

In 1973, the United States Supreme Court ruled that restricting a woman's right to an abortion violated her right to privacy. Over the next decade, the number of clinics offering amniocentesis for prenatal diagnosis skyrocketed.[27]

At the time, doctors recommended amniocentesis or chorionic villus biopsy for women over the age of 35 to diagnose Down syndrome and a few other, rarer, chromosomal anomalies. Conventional wisdom held that, for younger women, the added risk of miscarriage that was a consequence of amniocentesis outweighed the benefits of prenatal diagnosis. The availability of prenatal diagnosis forced all women—and their doctors—to think about whether or not they should take advantage of prenatal diagnosis. These new tests changed pregnancy into something different from what it had been before. In 1986, the sociologist Barbara Katz Rothman coined the term "tentative pregnancy" to describe the new experience of couples awaiting the results of prenatal diagnosis to decide whether to continue or terminate a pregnancy.

For those who chose to continue pregnancy, there would be another set of decisions about when, where, and how to deliver the baby. Some people advocated low-tech home births. Others recommended high-tech tertiary care centers equipped with the most sophisticated fetal monitors and with ready availability of surgical and neonatal care.

Whichever story is told about these profound changes, there is no denying that they have deeply affected the ways people think about sexuality, fertility, pregnancy, and childbirth. They have led many people to make individual and personal choices that, taken together, constitute trends that have contributed to the rise in the rate of preterm birth.

In this book we will explore and analyze many of these changes; we will suggest that they should alter the way we think about the fetus as a patient, about prenatal care, about labor and delivery, and about the ways we measure and evaluate outcomes for women and children.

2 Individual Decisions: A 34-Year-Old Pregnant Woman at 36 Weeks

Imagine this: You are a 34-year-old woman, pregnant for the first time. You got married when you were 30 but didn't want to have a baby right away. After about a year, you started trying to get pregnant. It was harder than you thought. A year and a half went by and still you were not pregnant.

You thought back to all those years when you had assiduously guarded against getting pregnant. Was that all wasted effort because you are actually incapable of conceiving? You remembered how you feared that any little slip would lead immediately and inevitably to an unwanted pregnancy. You remembered the panic caused by a slightly late period.

Now, the beginning of each period feels like a reminder that your body isn't working. You feel that damn biological clock ticking.

You find a wonderful obstetrician, a woman who is not much older than you and who seems very smart. One of your friends recommended her. The friend had also been having infertility problems. Your friend has a baby now, and says that she had a wonderful birth experience. The doctor does a thorough medical workup and recommends that you try to stimulate ovulation by taking the drug Clomid.

You worry about the possibility that you might end up with twins or triplets. You worry about the side effects—the bloating, the nausea, the mood swings, and the hot flashes. But you end up taking it. It works.

When you are around eight weeks, you see on the ultrasound image that there is just one tiny little fetus. You can see a head and what look like tiny little arms. You can even see a little heart beating. You feel tender, excited, and a little freaked out. A tiny creature is growing happily inside you. It is not apparent whether the fetus is a boy or a girl.

You really like your obstetrician but you are not sure that you want to give birth in a hospital. Another friend tells you about how she chose home birth with a midwife. The idea of a home birth seems intriguing and scary, natural and idiotic, rational and insane, all at the same time. You check out *Our Bodies, Our Blog* to see what the folks who brought you *Our Bodies, Ourselves* and started Boston's first midwifery program have to say about home birth. They offer statistics showing that, for low-risk women with uncomplicated pregnancies, it seems pretty safe. They criticize an article that appeared in *Time* magazine on September 4, 2010,[1] reviewing a study that claimed babies born at home were two or three times more likely to die than babies born in hospital.[2] That study summarized and aggregated data from 14 papers that had been published in the English-language, peer-reviewed literature. The findings: "Planned home births were associated with fewer maternal interventions including epidural analgesia, electronic fetal heart rate monitoring, episiotomy, and operative delivery. These women were less likely to experience lacerations, hemorrhage, and infections. Neonatal outcomes of planned home births revealed less frequent prematurity, low birthweight, and assisted newborn ventilation. Although planned home and hospital births exhibited similar perinatal mortality rates, planned home births were associated with significantly elevated neonatal mortality rates." The bloggers replied with a letter stating, "All reliable data on home birth midwifery in regulated and integrated systems like the Netherlands and Canada suggest that home birth is safe for the baby and associated with significant health benefits for the mother."[3] The letter was signed by more than a dozen doctors and researchers.

You start surfing the net for other information. You find that the American College of Obstetrics and Gynecology roundly and unambiguously condemns home birth, but that professional societies of obstetricians in Canada and Great Britain endorse it. You find personal birth stories from happy women who had their babies with the midwives at UCLA.[4] The women all say that they'd go to the midwives again. You also find "success stories" about obstetrician-attended hospital deliveries on the blogs and forums at www.obgyn.net, the ACOG website. These include stories written by women who developed serious complications during pregnancy or labor, whose babies were saved by swift and sometimes seemingly miraculous interventions by their physicians. The women are profoundly grateful to their doctors.

You wonder: are you a home-birth type of woman?

You decide to hedge your bets. You plan to deliver at a birthing center located inside a hospital. It is a lovely place. The prenatal care clinic waiting room is full of women at various stages of pregnancy. Some have that fatigued, nauseated first-trimester look. Others look calm and contented. You like to watch the look of concentration on their faces as their babies move or give a kick. Your baby seems to have a personality already. She has active days and quiet ones; she kicks more when you hear some genres of music than others. Your aunt said that your shape meant you were having a girl, and there are girls' names swirling through your head every day. You worry about whether you will be a good mom, and about whether your baby will love you. You think a lot about your own mom.

On some prenatal visits, you see the doctor. On others, you see the midwife. You think about writing a personal birth plan. But you don't.

You doctor recommends that you get something called a "quad screen." That's a new one on you. They tell you it is to see whether your baby is at risk for Down syndrome "or things like that." They do another ultrasound, too. You do another search to see what these tests are all about. A 2009 paper in the *American Journal of Obstetrics and Gynecology* informs you, "Women today have more options for Down syndrome screening than ever before, and the specific screening tests and diagnostic procedures continue to evolve."[5] That doesn't help you very much. Based upon your test results, the doctors say that the odds are very, very low that your baby could have Down syndrome or other chromosomal syndromes. You do not want them to tell you whether the baby is a boy or a girl.

You read baby books. You worry about having a preemie. You take your vitamins and stop drinking coffee, eating cheese and sushi, or changing cat litter. You go to every scheduled prenatal visit, even though not much seems to happen at each one. Mostly, they just take your blood pressure, weigh you, measure your belly, have you pee in a cup, and give you some advice. You could do all of that, it seems, by yourself at home. You have already seen the advice they give, online.

At 35 weeks, you start to have sharp abdominal pains. You wonder if it is early labor, but the pains are random, not regular. They are intense. They take your breath away and make you weak in the knees. You call the midwife. She listens carefully, asks some questions, and suggests that you lie down for the rest of the day and come into clinic the next morning. The next day, they do an ultrasound. The doctor looks worried, but says that the tests are basically reassuring. She wants you to come back in three days, rather than a week. Over the next few days, the sharp pains continue. It feels like perhaps the baby is moving and kicking a little less than the week before. At the next prenatal visit, the doctor says that the baby is not growing quite as much as expected. Your blood pressure is slightly elevated.

You discuss the options with your doctor. You could wait another few days. You could come into the hospital for closer fetal monitoring. They could induce delivery now. None of these options seems great. Still, none of the options seem terrible, either. You know that if your baby is born at 36 weeks, she will most likely be fine. The hospital has neonatologists and a NICU. You think, too, that if you just lie down and stop worrying, everything will probably be okay. The doctors do not think that it is urgent to deliver the baby. But every time you feel a twinge of abdominal pain, you worry. Then ten minutes go by without a kick. The thought of losing the baby now is unbearable. Tears roll slowly down your cheek.

What should you do? The decision you face is a very personal one. You have so much already invested in this pregnancy. You know this baby already. She has been talking to you for months, now, doing little somersaults and tai chi dances in your belly. She has been in your dreams most nights. All your ideas about an ideal birth, about your husband at your side, the roses on the windowsill, now suddenly seem irrelevant. You will do anything, or give up anything, to make sure your baby is okay. Your worst fear is that you could make a decision that will cause your baby to die before birth. But you can't figure out which choice is best.

The decision you face is also, oddly, political. It is about more than just you and your baby. Public health authorities, professional societies, litigators, insurance company executives, hospital administrators, the surgeon general of the United States, and the director of the March of Dimes, are all very interested in the decision you are about to make. These people, whom you have never met and will never meet, have a stake in the very personal decision that you and your doctor will make. They will be watching. They will collect data on you and your baby. They care about what you decide.

You just want to do what is best for your baby. It is your decision to make, granted to you by years of legal struggles to empower patients, buttressed by the philosophical arguments of a cadre of modern bioethicists, affirmed by feminists. You have the right to make decisions for yourself. You have the right to pursue your own happiness, to live a life based upon your own values. You are, after all, a competent adult, living in an individualistic, multicultural, multiethnic, non-theocratic, liberal, tolerant society, one that tolerates many different ideas about what is good and proper and will go to great lengths to protect your right to make judgments for yourself. You don't lose those rights just because you are a pregnant woman. Therefore, you could, if you wanted to, choose to have a cesarean section right now. You could choose to have labor induced right now. You have the hard-won right to decide when and where and how you want to have your baby.

But you don't feel particularly empowered. Instead, you feel various duties and obligations. First and foremost, you think of the health of your baby. You have already gone to great lengths and changed your own life in order to do what is best for the baby. You would do more. You would undergo a major abdominal operation if you thought it would help. You will bear the expenses of medical treatment (though you hope your insurance covers most of it). You want to do the right thing.

There are also some real constraints upon your freedom. Doctors and midwives do not have to help you if you ask them to do something that violates their conscience or their sense of professionalism. For example, if you decide that you want to deliver the baby right now, your doctor might not go along with your decision. She has her own duties and obligations. She could claim an obligation to do what is best for your baby, as well as for you, even if it is not what you want. If you wanted an abortion now, she would not go along with it. Your freedom ends where it violates her moral code, or the laws of the land. Your rights end where they impose unacceptable obligations upon others. The doctor, too, is a moral agent. You both live in a society with laws that govern the decisions that pregnant women can make at various stages of pregnancy.

You and your doctor may need to negotiate a plan that you can both live with. That negotiation can be described using the language of individual rights. It seems relatively straightforward and easy to understand, even if difficult to resolve.

More complicated questions arise when we recognize that there might be other stakeholders here besides you and your doctor. Does the surgeon general deserve a seat at the decision making table? What about the Centers for Disease Control? Or the U.S. Supreme Court? Your health insurance company? The March of Dimes? Your doctor's malpractice insurer? Your doctor's employer?

All of these third parties want to influence the decision that you and your doctor are about to make. The surgeon general and the Centers for Disease Control both have a mission to try to improve the health of the nation. They have both advocated policies to try to reduce the rate of preterm birth. They both want to decrease the number of preterm C-sections and inductions. So does the March of Dimes. Some doctors are incentivized by their employers to reduce these rates in their own practices. Yet preterm birth remains one of the most intractable public health problems of our time. Perhaps these third parties have a right to curtail the choices available to you, and to other pregnant women, just as they have the right to curtail the freedoms of people with influenza or tuberculosis under certain circumstances.

Your insurance company has obligations both to stockholders and to those who pay premiums to try to keep costs down, premiums low, and profits respectable. They can, under certain circumstances, limit the freedom of patients to make decisions. (Or at least they can limit what sorts of interventions they will pay for under certain circumstances.) If you choose to have a C-section, your health insurance rates might rise, just as your car insurance rates rise if you have an accident.

The American College of Obstetricians and Gynecologists (ACOG) also has a certain stake in the decision you make, and in your right to make that decision. Your freedom is, in a sense, their freedom. They want you to have the maximum freedom to make any decision that you want, no matter what it costs, as long as it does not force their members to violate their own moral codes. The Midwives Alliance of North America has a stake in your decision, too. They want to help you see childbirth "as a personal, intimate, internal, sexual and social experience to be shared in the environment and with the attendants a woman chooses" and to make sure that you and your partner have the right "to determine the most healing course of action when difficult situations arise."[6]

It is hard to tell just who is on your side and who is not, whose advice is self-serving and whose is selfless, who is most trustworthy to guide you in this difficult decision.

So there is one thing you can be sure of. You are not alone. But you feel lonely. And the decision seems to be yours alone. You must choose which facts to factor, whose advice to seek, and what trade-offs to make. You've always thought of yourself as an earthy, low-tech, home-birth type of woman. Now you are less sure.

In David Grossman's recent novel, *To the End of the Land,* the protagonist, Ora, finds herself thinking of the ways that she has fallen short as a feminist. She thinks that her life has become

an insult to women's lib, a stain on the neon glow that emanates from the books her friend Ariela insists on buying her, books she's never managed to read more than a few pages of, written by decisive, witty, opinionated women who use expressions like, "the duality of the clitoris as signifier and signified," or "the vagina as male-encoded deterministic space," which immediately activate in her feeble, characterless mind an interfering hum of machines and home appliances, blenders and vacuum cleaners and dishwashers—women who perceive her limp existence itself as a crude insult to them and their just struggle.[7]

Women who face decisions about childbirth may simultaneously feel that the decisions they make will somehow define them on the spectrum of feminism, and not want to think of those decisions as political. After all, in spite of the many compelling arguments about how obstetrics is unnatural, misogynist, profit-driven, and dangerous, most women continue to choose hospital births over home births, physicians over midwives, and high-tech births over natural ones. They seem to be disappointing not just feminists but also the public health authorities and health economists who see the number of interventions going up and the cost going up, as we all pay more for health care that does not make us any healthier, and call high-tech obstetrics a form of physician-induced demand that primarily serves the economic interests of the doctors, hospitals, and device manufacturers.

These experts must wonder how so many women can make the wrong decisions over and over again. Don't they see how their choices may lead to too many C-sections? Don't they know that their choices raise the cost of health care for us all without any compensatory benefit? Don't they see that they are choosing to increase—not decrease—the risks of morbidity and mortality for both themselves and their babies?

Of course, there is another story that can be told about these phenomena. It is possible that pregnant women are, in fact, smarter than all the experts. It is possible that they understand the arguments, evaluate the evidence, consider the alternatives, and then make wise decisions for themselves and their babies based on their own understanding of the risks, benefits, costs, and consequences of one choice compared to another. It is possible that all of these individual decisions, however flawed and problematic in the aggregate, are, in fact, the best decisions that could be made by the individuals in the circumstances. Perhaps pregnant women—and their doctors—have a more complete understanding than all the public health authorities, health economists, and feminists put together.

Your abdominal pain is not getting any better. It doesn't seem to be getting any worse. Your mood, though, is terrible. You are in a no-win situation. Your doctor is still nondirective in her counseling. She gives you two choices—she can continue monitoring you and your baby and, if things get worse, intervene. Or she can try to induce delivery now with Pitocin and, if that fails, do a C-section. With that option, your baby will be born slightly preterm. You wish that somebody would give you a balance sheet with the facts. What exactly is the risk, if you decide to continue the pregnancy rather than induce labor now?

3   Stillbirth

The biggest risk of not doing a C-section, of waiting and monitoring, is that your baby will die in the womb. The reason why doctors sometimes recommend C-sections, even for preterm babies, is to avoid that risk. It is much easier to monitor and care for a baby born at 36 weeks in the NICU than it is to monitor a 36 week fetus in the womb. But how high is the risk of a stillbirth at this point in pregnancy?

There are probably more than a million fetal deaths per year in the United States.[1] That number is not very helpful in your situation. Most fetal deaths occur very early in pregnancy and are not actually reported or tracked. As a result, the exact number of fetal deaths is an estimate. It is based on data from retrospective surveys that ask women if they were pregnant in the last year and, if so, what was the outcome of the pregnancy. Based upon one such survey of about 12,000 Americans, the National Survey for Family Growth, Ventura and colleagues estimated that in 2005 there were 6,408,000 pregnancies in the United States. These resulted in 4.14 million live births, 1.21 million induced abortions, and 1.06 million fetal deaths.[2] That number—a million fetal deaths—is likely an underestimate, since women who did not yet know they were pregnant are often unaware of early fetal loss. But that number is also not relevant to the situation of a woman at 36 weeks.

Most states require doctors to report fetal deaths that occur after 20 weeks of gestation, which is halfway through the second trimester. Those numbers are more relevant to your situation. But they are also somewhat inaccurate, because reporting criteria vary from state to state. Some states follow the recommendations of the American College of Obstetrics and Gynecology and the World Health Organization to report fetal death only after 22 weeks of gestation or if the fetus weighs more than 500 grams (about one pound). Other states use 20 weeks of gestation as the cutoff for reporting and do not have criteria for fetal weight.

The National Center for Health Statistics aggregates states' reports of fetal deaths after 20 weeks of gestation going back to the early 1980s. They divide fetal deaths into two categories— early and late. Early fetal deaths are those that occur between 20 and 27 weeks of gestation. Late fetal deaths are those that occur at 28 weeks or later. Note, again, that nobody keeps track of fetal deaths before 20 weeks of gestation. By these categories, you would be in the latter category. If your baby died in the womb now, it would be a "late" fetal death.

There were 25,894 reported fetal deaths after 20 weeks of gestation in the United States in 2005.[3] About half of these occurred before and half after 27 weeks of gestation.

Some groups of women are at higher risk for a fetal death than others. Fetal mortality rates are highest in women over the age of 35. For those women, 9 out of every 1000 pregnancies ended in a stillbirth after 20 weeks of gestation. By comparison, the number was only 5.7 per 1000 for women 20 to 34 years of age. Among teenagers, 7.5 out of every 1000 pregnancies end in stillbirth. Put another way, women 35 to 39 years of age are 1.9 times as likely as women under 30 to have a fetal demise. Things get worse for women over 40. They are 2.7 times as likely as women under 30 to lose a baby this way.[4] You are 34, so you might be more like the 35- to 39-year-olds than the 20- to 34-year-olds. So your chance of stillbirth is probably less than one percent. And you are married, white, and carrying a singleton. All of those things decrease the chances that you will have a stillborn baby. Married women have lower reported fetal death rates than unmarried women. Blacks have higher rates than other racial and ethnic groups. Twins and other multiples are at higher risk. Male fetuses are more likely to die than female fetuses, for reasons nobody can explain. You also need to consider medical risk factors. Congenital anomalies of the fetus account for 25% to 35% of stillbirths.[5] But your ultrasound exam was normal. Maternal infections, including viral, bacterial, and protozoal infections, account for another 10% to 25% of all fetal deaths.[6] Women with diabetes, hypertension, or obesity are more likely to have a stillbirth than women without those problems.[7] You are in the clear on these matters. But many cases of stillbirth occur with no risk factors and no explanation. They just happen.[8] So, if you factor in all those things, your risk of a stillbirth probably drops to less than one half of one percent.

Things have been getting better over the last thirty years. Fetal death rates have been steadily dropping since the mid-1980s. In 1985, 7.83 of every 1,000 pregnancies ended in stillbirth. By 2004, the rate had fallen by 20%, to 6.20 in 1,000. And most of the decline has been in late fetal deaths, those after 27 weeks of gestation, where the rate has fallen nearly 40%, from 4.95 to 3.09 per 1,000.[9] These trends are shown in figure 3.1.

Much of the decline can be attributed to improved access to prenatal care, leading to better fetal screening and the early

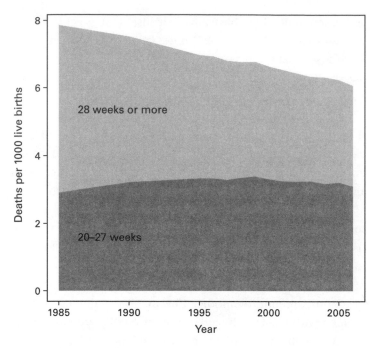

Figure 3.1
Early and late fetal mortality rates in the United States, 1990–2005. Data
from the National Vital Statistics Service; MacDorman MF et al. Fetal and
perinatal mortality, United States, 2006. National vital statistics reports;
vol 60 no 8. http://www.cdc.gov/nchs/data/nvsr/nvsr60/nvsr60_08.pdf.

diagnosis of pregnancy problems. Prevention and treatment of
perinatal infections and effective treatment of maternal medical conditions such as diabetes and chronic hypertension all are
thought to contribute to improved fetal survival.[10]

But consider this: the longer you wait to deliver the baby, the
higher the chance of a stillbirth. Fetal death rates are highest
early in pregnancy, lowest between 26 and 34 weeks of gestation,

and then rise sharply after 36 weeks. This is particularly true for women who are older than 35. Fretts calculated that delivery of all babies at 39 weeks of gestational age would prevent 2 fetal deaths for every 1000 living fetuses at 39 weeks. This would translate into the prevention of as many as 6,000 intrauterine fetal deaths in the United States annually.[11] Nobody has done such a calculation on deliveries at 36 or 37 weeks or for 34-year-olds in particular. Those are the numbers that you would really like to know.

So the data on your risk of having a stillbirth are not conclusive. To apply those statistics to your situation, you would need to place yourself on the various risk curves. You are just about the age where the risk of a stillborn starts going up. And you are at about 36 weeks of gestation, the time of pregnancy when the likelihood of stillbirth starts to increase. Your overall health has been good, you're not obese, and you don't have diabetes. You are white, married, and have no prior history of a preterm birth or a stillbirth. Statistically speaking, these factors would all lower the chances of stillbirth. You don't know if your baby is male or female. It seems that the overall risk is quite low, somewhere between 1 in 200 and 1 in 1,000. But it will slowly rise with each passing day. And someone will be the one in 200 or the one in 1,000.

The slow, steady rise in stillbirth rates in the final weeks of pregnancy creates one of the most difficult dilemmas facing obstetricians and their patients today. When is it safer to deliver the baby early than it is to continue the pregnancy? If you delivered the baby now, what problems would she or could she have?

4   Late Preterm Birth

You try to learn about the risks to the baby of being born at 35 or 36 weeks of gestation rather than going to full term. You quickly find that there is a lot of debate about the best thing to do and about the relative risks of continuing the pregnancy or inducing delivery. The confusion comes, in part, because it is impossible to do the rigorous scientific studies that could definitively answer the questions about risks and benefits. For such studies to be done, women like you would have to be *randomly* assigned to have a C-section or to waiting for natural labor to begin. Then, we could compare the results and really know which was the better approach, overall. That study will never happen because nobody would let a flip of a coin decide which women would get a C-section and which women would continue their pregnancies while each little fetal heart rate abnormality is carefully noted on the monitor. Without the random assignment, differences in outcomes for the early C-sections versus others could be due to myriad differences between the mothers and babies that led to different choices. And so, doctors and scientists pore over the retrospective data, trying to figure out which babies really needed to be delivered early and which babies would have been better off with another week in the womb.

The first problem is to determine precisely—and then classify—the baby's gestational age at delivery. The classification of births by gestational age is complicated and, of late, has become politically fraught as well. For decades, the duration of pregnancy (and thus the gestational age of the fetus) was defined in relationship to the onset of a woman's last menstrual period (LMP). Counting from that day, a full-term pregnancy was defined as one that lasted from 37 weeks and 0 days (commonly denoted by doctors as 37/0) until 41 weeks and 6 days (denoted 41/6). Deliveries before 37 weeks after the first day of the LMP were considered preterm. Deliveries at 42 weeks or more were considered post-term.

The date of the LMP was used not because it was completely accurate but because it was something a woman actually knew. The actual date of conception is much harder to determine. New technologies allow home ovulation testing. These might be used to establish the date of conception with a little more precision for some women. Home pregnancy testing is also getting more and more accurate, but even today, pregnancy tests do not generally turn positive until two weeks after conception occurs.

Another way to determine gestational age is with fetal ultrasound. Ultrasound dating relies on measurement of certain body dimensions in the fetus. In the first trimester, the "crown-rump length" can be used to establish accurate gestational age within 3 to 5 days.[1] In the second trimester, head circumference is another measurement that allows estimation of gestation age. Both have a margin of error of 3 to 5 days, but both allow estimates of gestational age that are generally more accurate than those determined by recollection of the LMP. Comparisons of ultrasound with dating by LMP show that the latter is likely to overestimate the true gestational age by about one day.[2]

Why does a day or two matter? Two reasons. First, gestational age is used to estimate risk, and levels of risk are used to make clinical decisions. If your baby is preterm, doctors will be less likely to recommend a C-section than if your baby is full-term. So the classification of gestational age may determine what treatment you should choose. The second reason is more relevant to epidemiology and health policy. Our public health system is constantly measuring the rate of preterm birth and trying to reduce it. As noted above, however, the rate remains quite high. One reason that our measured rates of preterm birth have risen may be that doctors use ultrasound more than they used to. Since ultrasound is more accurate and thus more likely to date a pregnancy as having begun later, it tends to lead to assignment of lower gestational age. This, of course, does not represent a real rise in the preterm birth rate. It is, instead, just a recognition that we used to underestimate that rate because, using the LMP method, we were overestimating gestational age.

The use of ultrasound dating rather than dating based on LMP will also mean that, if doctors are waiting until a baby reaches a specific gestational age such as 37 weeks before inducing delivery in a case like yours, they will wait a little longer. And, as we showed above, the likelihood of a stillbirth, while low, will rise with each passing day.

There is also hot debate about whether the definitions that have traditionally been used to define a birth as preterm, term, or postterm are accurate, useful, or in need of revision. In 2012, a group of pediatricians, obstetricians, epidemiologists, and policy makers from around the world gathered in Bethesda, Maryland, to examine whether our system for classifying preterm, term, and postterm should be changed.[3] This consensus conference began by asking what those classifications are used for. They noted that one of the main uses of the classification is as a measure of mortality risk. Infant mortality is higher for babies born preterm or post-term than for babies born at term. But those mortality differences are only useful if the gestational age assignments upon which they are based are accurate. More recent data allows those prognostic indicators to be fine-tuned. It turns out that infant mortality and morbidity is lower for babies born at 39 or 40 weeks than it is for babies born at 37, 38, or 41 weeks. Thus, even for babies conventionally grouped together as "term" babies, there are more optimum and less optimum days for delivery.

The consensus conference in Bethesda suggested that the traditional classification criteria, by which a baby born between 37 and 42 weeks would be considered a "term" baby, was inadequate. Instead, they suggested that a baby born at 37 or 38 weeks be considered "early term," a baby born at 39 or 40 weeks be considered term, and a baby born at 41 weeks be considered "late term." Such classifications seem long overdue. What may sound like splitting hairs would actually allow subtle but real distinctions to be made that could affect the way outcomes are predicted, shaping both clinical practice and public policy.

After all, the policy debate about preterm birth is driven by the number of births that fall into arbitrarily defined categories. Calculating gestational age on the basis of ultrasound rather than LMP might lead to a rise in the recorded rate of preterm birth, even though nothing had actually changed except the way certain births were categorized.

Much of the data we have on outcomes is based upon current categories. Thus, a baby born at 34 through 36 weeks of gestation is considered a "late preterm" birth. This classification scheme, however, overlooks differences between babies born at 34, 35, and 36 weeks. It also suggests complacency about a 37-week delivery that might be unwarranted. Such distinctions might be crucial for your decision about whether or not to induce delivery now. You would like a more nuanced prognosis than current numbers can provide. You are not the only one who has a problem here. The assignment of babies to one or another category can lead policy makers to misleading assessments of the nature of the problems associated with preterm birth. A central theme of this book is that the rise in preterm births is usually viewed as a major public health problem. But a rise in the percentage of babies born two days early is very different from a rise in the percentage of babies born two weeks or two months early. As it turns out, almost all of the rise in preterm births over the last 25 years has been in late preterm births. Most of it is accounted for by babies born between 34 and 36 weeks of gestation. Over those years, the rate of preterm birth at 32 to 33 weeks increased only slightly. The rate of preterm birth at less than 32 weeks has stayed stubbornly the same. The graph in figure 4.1 illustrates this trend, showing both the increase, and the recent fall, in the preterm birth rate at various gestational ages.

This situation presents a dilemma for clinicians and policy makers. Early preterm births are the most dangerous in terms of infant mortality or lifelong chronic illness for babies who survive. When most people hear the term "preterm," they likely picture tiny early preterm babies. Arguably, policy efforts should focus more on those early preterm births. But late preterm births are where the action is in terms of rising rates. Efforts to lower rates of preterm birth that address the late preterm births are the ones most likely to be successful; but those efforts will have the least impact on infant mortality. By contrast, efforts to lower the rate of early preterm birth would, if successful, have the greatest

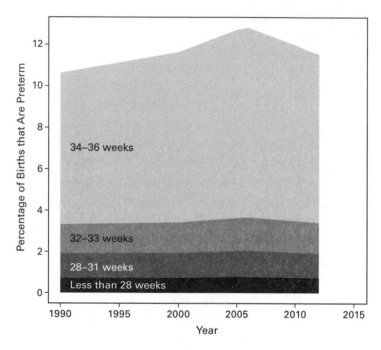

Figure 4.1
Preterm birth rates at different gestational ages in the United States, 1990–2012. Source of data: Martin JA, Hamilton BE, Osterman MJK, Curtin SC, Mathews TJ. Births: Final data for 2012. National vital statistics reports; vol 62 no 9. Hyattsville, MD: National Center for Health Statistics; 2013. http://www.cdc.gov/nchs/data/nvsr/nvsr62/nvsr62_09.pdf.

impact on infant mortality. But, to date, no interventions have had any effect whatsoever on the rate of early preterm birth.

Policy makers have focused on late preterm births because those are the ones that we seem to be able to do something about. As we shall show below, many late preterm births are medically induced, either by pharmacological induction of labor or by C-section. Some, perhaps many, of those medical inductions may be unnecessary. If obstetricians could lower the rate of unnecessary inductions and C-sections, they could lower the rate of late preterm birth, and we assume that that will also improve the health of women and their babies. The problem with that assumption, of course, is the problem you face as you lie there in the examining room of the labor and delivery suite with painful abdominal cramps and some abnormalities on the fetal heart rate monitor. How do we know which medically induced preterm births are unnecessary, and thus which babies would be better off staying in the womb than being delivered early?

There are risks to early delivery in the "late preterm" weeks. A number of studies have tried to quantify those risks. The studies are difficult to interpret, however, because there are at least three groups of such babies and, for most of the data studied, it is impossible to be sure which group is most appropriate for a particular baby. One group is the group babies whose mothers first went into preterm labor spontaneously, but the labor was not progressing and they went on to receive either Pitocin to accelerate labor or a C-section. Another group consists of those babies who were delivered early because there were strong indications of problems with the pregnancy or signs of fetal distress. The final group is women who want to have an early delivery. They may want this for many reasons. Some births do not fall neatly into one of these groups, and it is not always clear from birth records which birth ought to be assigned to which group. The key question is this: Do babies who are born early have more problems because they were born early? Or are babies (or pregnancies) with problems more likely to end up with a preterm delivery? In other words, is the preterm birth the cause of problems or the result of the problems?

Here are some examples of the types of studies that try to tease out the risks of early delivery and to separate those risks from whatever problems may have led to the early delivery. Bird and colleagues studied birth outcomes for 5188 singleton babies, all without birth defects noted prenatally, who were born at 34 to 36 weeks of gestation and compared them with 15,303 babies born at term.[4] The researchers matched the preterm babies to the term babies by infant, maternal, and clinical characteristics to make the two comparison groups as similar as possible with respect to those factors that might have predicted preterm birth, in order to separately predict problems for the baby's health. They found that the preterm babies were more likely to have respiratory distress, to require mechanical ventilation, and to have low blood sugar. Those babies also had more medical problems during the first year of life, leading to health expenditures that were five times higher than those for matched babies born at term. Even with matching, however, the researchers couldn't tease out the independent effect of fetal distress. More of the babies born early had some signs of fetal distress before their delivery. The fetal distress may have been what led to the decision to deliver the baby early. Thus, the early delivery may not have been so much the cause of the later problems as a "marker" of the underlying health issues that went on to cause problems down the road.

Still, such studies suggest that early delivery, by itself, does cause problems. A report from the American Academy of Pediatrics that reviews a number of such studies concludes that late preterm babies have higher risks of feeding difficulties, jaundice, respiratory distress, and hypoglycemia compared to term babies.[5] They are more likely than term babies to be admitted to the NICU, to be evaluated for sepsis, and to receive intravenous antibiotics. During the initial birth hospitalization, late preterm infants are 4 times more likely than term infants to have at least one medical condition diagnosed and 3.5 times more likely to have two or more conditions diagnosed.[6] As a result of all these complications, late preterm babies have higher infant mortality risk than term babies.[7]

Such studies and such statistics are tricky to interpret, of course, because they often do not and cannot distinguish among the various reasons for preterm delivery. As the American Academy of Pediatrics report notes,

It is important to understand why these infants are being born early... Fetuses considered to be at risk of stillbirth, including those with intrauterine growth restriction, fetal anomalies, and intrapartum asphyxia, may be identified earlier, which results in more deliveries at 34 to 36 weeks' gestation. It is important to note that the increased intensity of care provided to pregnant women has been accompanied by significant reductions in stillbirths, perinatal mortality, and births beyond 40 weeks' gestation.

Some of the morbidity and mortality seems to be due to cesarean delivery alone. Even term babies who are delivered by elective C-section have higher rates of respiratory distress, hypoglycemia, and NICU admission.[8,9] But, again, there are always ambiguities about why the C-section was elected, so it is hard to know how much of the increased morbidity and mortality among late preterm births is due to the C-section as opposed to the medical conditions that led to the C-section.[10] Again, we face the causation question. Are babies who are delivered by C-section at higher risk because they are delivered by C-section? Or are babies who are having problems the ones who get delivered by C-section?

Induced early delivery has risks not just for your baby but also for you. If you try to induce delivery and it does not work, you will likely end up having a C-section. Women who have

C-sections are at increased risk for infection, blood clots, bowel problems, and chronic abdominal pain. C-sections may lead to complications in future pregnancies, including uterine rupture or severe bleeding during labor and delivery. On the other hand, there may also be benefits to having a C-section. Women who have C-sections are less likely to have incontinence or other pelvic problems after pregnancy.[11] We will present more detailed data about C-sections in the next chapter.

You do not know how to balance all the risks and benefits. You are glad to have all this data, but it just raises more questions. Each new bit of data makes you less certain of what to do. Knowledge is supposed to empower you, but you feel helpless and confused in the face of the conflicting, imprecise data. How are you supposed to think about a degree of risk like 1 out of 200? Is that a high risk or a low risk?

You have to make a decision. You want to make the decision based on the facts. But the facts just make you more uncertain. Maybe you should just trust your doctor and do whatever she says.

But that raises another set of concerns. Can you trust her to do what is best for you? Some critics of obstetrics claim that doctors recommend C-sections not because the operations are medically necessary but because, by doing more C-sections, the doctors make more money or are less likely to be sued. Some claim that doctors do them in order to have more control over their time and their work environment. As is the case for many of the issues we discuss in this book, there is a lot of data and analysis devoted to figuring out whether or to what degree such claims are true. Such studies try to determine just how many C-sections are done for bona fide medical indications and how many are the result of a phenomenon that economists have called "physician-induced demand." The next chapter will review some of that data.

5   Are There Too Many C-sections?

Doctors in the United States perform a lot of C-sections. In 2013, there were almost 1.3 million C-sections.[1] That is more than 3,500 per day, or about one every 20 seconds. In 2012, one-third of all deliveries in the United States were by C-section. The C-section rate in the United States has been rising steadily since the late 1990s. In 1970, only 5.1% of deliveries in the United States were by C-section. By 1980, C-sections were performed in 16% of all deliveries. The rate leveled off in the 1980s and then began to rise once again in the 1990s. By 2011, C-sections were performed in 33% of deliveries in the United States.[2] The trend is shown in figure 5.1, which shows the proportion of births by C-section in the United States between 1991 and 2007. The rate has continued to hover close to 33% for the last few years.

One might expect that the rise in C-sections would have occurred primarily among women thought to be at higher risk for pregnancy problems. That does not seem to be the case. Over the last few decades, the rate of C-sections rose equally among women in all age groups and all racial groups. The increase occurred for women with private health insurance, public health insurance, or no health insurance. C-section rates rose just as

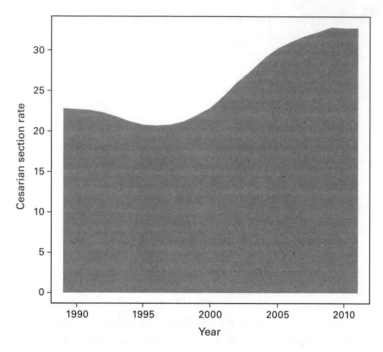

Figure 5.1
Cesarean delivery rate in the United States, 1991–2011. Data from Martin JA et al., Births: Final data for 2012. National vital statistics reports; vol 62 no 9. http://www.cdc.gov/nchs/data/nvsr/nvsr62/nvsr62_09.pdf.

fast among women with no identifiable risk factors for pregnancy problems as among women with identifiable risk factors.[3] Rates rose at about the same pace for preterm babies and for term babies.

The Surgeon General has repeatedly called for fewer C-sections. As with calls to lower the rate of preterm birth, these exhortations have had little effect. In the report issued in the early 1990s, *Healthy People 2000*, the surgeon general urged that the C-section rate be kept below 15% of all deliveries.[4] Over the next decade it rose to 21%. *Healthy People 2010*, issued in 2001, again called for a rate of 15%.[5] Over the next few years, the rate rose to 33%.

In most cases, there is some plausible reason why a C-section is performed. Your case might be a typical one. Your baby is moving a little less. You are 34 years old. You are having abdominal pain. These are all reasons to worry that your baby might be in trouble. They are all reasons why your doctor wants to monitor you more closely, to be attentive to the possibility that your baby may be in trouble. But is a C-section really necessary? Will it decrease the risk that your pregnancy will end in a stillbirth? Or will it just increase the risk to you: the risk of undergoing a surgical procedure that may lead to a life-threatening infection, one that may make it harder for you to get pregnant a second time or may lead to a uterine rupture if you ever try to deliver vaginally in a future pregnancy? What are the chances of each of these outcomes? Nobody knows for sure. People can cite statistics, but the statistics in this situation only provide a quantitative measure of uncertainty, rather than a precise prediction of what will happen to any individual patient. For you, the likelihood of a good outcome is much higher than the likelihood of a bad outcome. But the psychological cost of a bad outcome, should one occur, is likely more than you want to pay.

When experts review the medical records for all C-sections, they find tremendous variation in the rate of C-sections without any apparent related difference in outcomes. For example, Kozhimannil and colleagues studied all births at 593 different hospitals in 2009 throughout the United States. All of the hospitals had more than 100 deliveries that year. These researchers found that C-section rates varied tenfold. In some hospitals, only 7.1% of deliveries were by C-section. In others, nearly 70% were.

The rates were higher for women with known risk factors for pregnancy problems. But even for women with lower-risk pregnancies (that is, women not delivering preterm, without a prior C-section, and not presenting with the fetus in a difficult position), in which more limited variation might be expected, C-section rates varied by a factor of 15, from 2.4% to 36.5%.[6] That is, there was more variation among hospitals for low risk women than for the overall population. The rates were, on average, similar (and similarly variable) at urban versus rural hospitals, at small versus large hospitals, and at teaching versus non-teaching hospitals. There was no evidence that the outcomes for babies were better at the hospitals with the higher C-section rates.

The variation in C-section rates is similar to the variation in rates of many other medical and surgical interventions.[7] Such variation has been a focus of health services research. Many explanations have been offered for these seemingly irrational and idiosyncratic variations in practice. All of them acknowledge that there are limits to approaches that aim to rationalize or standardize medical care. As one commentary pointedly asked, "What is the role of clinical judgment in the face of inadequate research evidence and legitimate physician and patient preferences?"[8]

The most cynical explanation for the rising rate of C-sections is that doctors do it for the money. This is not implausible. After all, physicians are in a unique position to advance their own economic interests. They have special expertise. Patients trust them. Sure, physicians promise to use their expertise to do what is best for patients. But it is not always completely clear what is best for patients. In such situations, when one medically defensible choice leads to much more income for doctors than another, it is plausible that doctors will favor the more lucrative choice.

Doctors, after all, are only human. They might use their unique position of power and influence to create what may seem to be a win-win situation by steering patients toward procedures that may help the patients and certainly put more money in the doctors' pockets.[9]

Health economists have studied patterns in the use of C-sections to see if they can find evidence that the operations are motivated by physicians' desire to increase their own income. It turns out to be a phenomenon that is much easier to imagine than it is to document. Economists have to be very creative in trying to show that doctors' practice variations are motivated by profits.

Gruber and Owings designed a fascinating study based upon the following phenomena, assumptions, and hypotheses.[10] They noted that fertility rates declined in the United States between 1970 and 1982. At the same time, they observed, the number of practicing obstetricians in different states either stayed the same or increased. Thus, each obstetrician would have fewer opportunities to deliver babies in 1982 than in 1970. If all else stayed equal, these economists hypothesized, then obstetricians' incomes should have fallen. They calculated that a 10% decline in the fertility rate would lead to a 5% drop in the income of obstetricians if the doctors did not change their practices by doing more costly procedures.

Further, and luckily, these researchers also noted that the fall in fertility rates was different in different states. Thus, for example, in North Carolina, fertility rates dropped from 1.93 births per 100 women of childbearing age to 1.42 per 100 between 1970 and 1982, a 26% decline. This would have led to a 13% drop in income. In Kansas, during those same years, the fertility rate fell for a few years but then quickly rose back to its 1970 level of about 1.7 per 100. Gruber and Owens tested the assumption that doctors would try to preserve their income. Were that assumption true, they predicted that C-section rates should have risen more in North Carolina (or other states that saw similar fertility declines) than in states like Kansas that did not see lower fertility. That is what they found. "A fall in the fertility rate of 10% is associated with an increase in the likelihood of cesarean delivery of .97 percentage points." A plausible explanation is that doctors steered patients toward decisions that would preserve the doctors' income. Gruber and Owens noted, however, that the change was not as dramatic as they would have predicted. "A one percentage point rise in cesarean utilization translates to 1.68 more cesarean deliveries per year, or…an income rise of only 0.5%." This was nowhere near enough to make up for the loss of income associated with the decreased fertility rate.

They summarize their results as follows: "Our basic findings are supportive of the hypothesis that ob/gyns responded to falling fertility in this era by performing more cesarean section deliveries. The estimated response is small, however, relative to the shock to ob/gyn income, and our finding implies that the general fertility decrease during this era can explain only a small part of the overall growth in cesarean utilization."

Other studies have found similar results. For example, Tussing and Wojtowycz tried to determine whether doctors change their behavior based upon their own interests, rather than those of the patient.[11] They examined three different external influences—fear of malpractice litigation, desire for more income, and desire for more convenient delivery times—to see whether these factors influenced doctors' decisions about C-sections.

They "failed to find much support for the idea that obstetricians perform cesareans to enrich themselves from the additional fee income." In fact, they found a negative correlation between the ratio of obstetricians to fertile females and the C-section rate. They did find that the busiest doctors tended to do more C-sections than doctors who were less busy. They note, "One possible explanation is that busy doctors perform more cesarean sections to manage their time; and obstetricians and others who deliver babies are more likely to be busy where there is a low ratio of obstetricians to fertile females." This would be a different sort of physician-induced demand, one based not on the goal of maximizing income but, instead, on the goal of preserving free time.

In a follow-up study, these same researchers focused on the effect of the fear of malpractice accusations. In order to examine the effect of malpractice fears, they compared C-section rates among doctors in counties that had different rates of malpractice litigation against obstetricians. Such a comparison does not, strictly speaking, measure doctors' fears—it may be a measure of doctors' perceptions of the realities of the communities in which they practice. But the researchers found a correlation. "Of an overall C-section rate of 27.6% in the data set, fear of malpractice accounts for an estimated 6.6 percentage points, of which 4.4 percentage points reflect a direct effect, and the remaining 2.2 percentage points reflect the effect of malpractice exposure on the use of electronic fetal monitoring and, directly and indirectly, the diagnosis of fetal distress."[12]

It is also possible, of course, that malpractice litigation follows bad outcomes and that C-sections reduce the rate of bad outcomes.

Malpractice litigation might have influenced physicians in another way, too. Obstetricians' incomes go down when malpractice premiums rise. Thus, if physicians induce demand for more lucrative services because their income is falling, then rising malpractice premiums might be expected to have an impact on obstetricians' decisions similar to that of decreasing fertility rates. Benedetti and colleagues studied this hypothesis by surveying obstetricians, rural and urban family physicians, and midwives in Washington State about their practice changes in relation to their malpractice insurance premiums. They found that, between 2002 and 2004, malpractice premiums for obstetricians rose by 61%. These doctors were asked how they responded to the rapid rise in malpractice premiums. Doctors reported that they raised cash by taking out loans or selling assets, and that their incomes dropped. They did not report deliberate or conscious changes in practice patterns as a result of rising insurance premiums. Nevertheless, over these years, their practice patterns did change. Specifically, they increased the number of deliveries they attended and their C-section rates. They decreased the number of high-risk cases in their practices. The authors were cautious in their conclusions about rising C-section rates: "Whether this change was related to defensive medical practice, renewed concerns about the safety of vaginal birth after cesarean delivery, or hospital policy (e.g., no vaginal birth after cesarean deliveries without an in-hospital anesthesiologist throughout labor) cannot be determined from this survey."[13]

This study suggests that there are complex relationships among economic incentives and disincentives for providers of obstetric services. C-sections may be more lucrative in themselves than vaginal deliveries. They may also lower the risk of lawsuit. But high-risk deliveries, in which C-sections may be more likely, also increase the risk of being sued. Doctors seemed to respond to the higher cost of malpractice in a number of ways—accepting lower income, working harder, and changing many aspects of their practice.

In a follow-up study, Baldwin and colleagues examined the relationship between obstetric practices and actual malpractice lawsuits in Washington State. Their conclusion: "After controlling for patient, physician, and sociodemographic characteristics, we found no difference in prenatal resource use or cesarean delivery rate for low-risk patients between physicians with more and less exposure to malpractice claims."[14] In a similar study from Florida, Entman and colleagues divided Florida's obstetricians into groups according to their history of being sued. They had a group of doctors who were sued more frequently than others, a group with an average number of suits, a lower than average group, and a group with no lawsuits at all. They found no differences among any of the groups in the frequency with which they performed C-sections (or in any other measure of quality care.)[15] On the other hand, Localio and colleagues found a positive association between C-section rates at hospitals and the average malpractice premium paid by doctors who practiced at those hospitals; that is, when one was higher the other also tended to be higher.[16] Similarly, Dubay and colleagues used national birth certificate data to study obstetricians from around the country. They found some evidence of defensive medicine but not much: "The study provides evidence that physicians practice defensive medicine in obstetrics but that the impact of increased cesarean sections that results from malpractice fears on total obstetric care costs is small."[17]

A third possible economic incentive for doctors to recommend C-sections, in addition to the desire for more income or the desire to avoid litigation, could be that they just want more control of their time. In economic jargon, there is a "market" in leisure time. Some studies suggest that doctors perform more C-sections so that they will be able to get home from work earlier or be less likely to be called in during the night. Tussing and Wojtowycz examined this and concluded that "obstetricians occasionally perform cesarean sections to manage their time, which does represent a form of economic self-interest."

Another way to try to measure the effect of doctors' self-interest on C-section rates is to analyze the decisions of salaried doctors in prepaid group practices. They do not make any more money by doing more C-sections. In fact, in some practices, they may even be incentivized not to do C-sections since, in such a practice model, higher-cost treatments would decrease profit margins. Spetz and colleagues analyzed the timing of C-section deliveries for patients in group-model health maintenance organizations (HMOs) compared to other patients. They found that C-sections were, in fact, performed less often for patients in the group-model HMO. They also found that C-sections were done at all hours of the day or night in the HMO patients, whereas in the comparison group they were more likely to be performed in the evening hours. The higher rate of C-sections in the evening hours, they thought, might be a result of doctors' reluctance to stay up all night waiting for labor to progress. They concluded that because of the structure of financial incentives, group-model HMOs "may be better able to guide physician practice, and they might provide staff support to physicians so there is less leisure-based incentive to perform cesarean sections."[18]

A final bit of complexity in the relationship between rising C-section rates and economic incentives is the fact that rates are rising in most other countries. In Britain, the C-section rate rose from 18% in 1997 to 22% in 2000.[19] Canada saw a similar rise.[20] Among eight countries of Latin America, C-section rates range from 33% to 51%.[21] These countries have very different models of health-care financing. In some countries, doctors make more money by performing more C-sections; in others, they do not. But the rate is rising everywhere. And the medical malpractice climate in other countries is completely different.

The overall conclusion from these studies is that doctors' motives are not completely pure, but they are less contaminated by self-interest than some of the harshest critics suggest. Doctors are influenced by their own economic interest, they have an interest in maximizing their leisure time, and they want to avoid malpractice suits. But these factors play less of a role in the rising rate of C-sections than some other, less well-understood factors.

C-sections are among those medical procedures whose goal is to prevent fatal outcomes, but which are done in situations where no good diagnostic tests can precisely predict which patients are at risk for those bad outcomes. There are other situations like this. Pediatricians do many lumbar punctures in order to rule out meningitis. The great majority of the lumbar punctures are negative. But it is judged that the risks of a lumbar puncture are low enough, and the consequences of missing a diagnosis of meningitis are high enough, that a high ratio of negative tests to positive ones is appropriate. The same has long been true of appendectomies for suspected appendicitis, although improved imaging has recently allowed doctors to more accurately diagnose or rule out appendicitis. Nevertheless, about 5% to 10% of operations for suspected appendicitis still reveal a normal appendix.[22] Such operations could, in retrospect, be called unnecessary. In these situations, as with C-sections, we assume that the invasive procedure is beneficial—allowing us to save a life that would otherwise have been lost or to prevent more serious complications—and that those benefits outweigh the risks of the procedure. If we could more precisely define the population at risk of a bad outcome, we would do fewer procedures.

But it is difficult to identify the boundary between appropriate caution and overuse. The key difference between C-sections and other clinical situations (such as in the meningitis or appendicitis examples above) is that, in most other situations we will eventually know whether the concern that led to the invasive procedure was warranted or not. That is, we find out whether a patient had meningitis or appendicitis, and so we know whether or not the pre-procedure diagnosis was correct. With C-sections, we cannot know what the outcome would have been had the procedure not been performed. So it is harder to determine just which C-sections were necessary or unnecessary.

Your own doctor seems to be reluctant to recommend a C-section, even though it might, for all the reasons noted above, be in her own interest to do so. You are not sure how to interpret her reluctance. Perhaps she is valiantly struggling against the various temptations to perform an unnecessary C-section. Or she might be in a practice group that incentivizes her to keep her C-section rate low (an incentive her patients would never know about). While you certainly do not want an unnecessary C-section, you don't want the decision to be driven by anything other than an assessment of your well-being and the well-being of your baby. Overall, you trust both her judgment and her ethics. But there are other reasons, deeper philosophical reasons, why her advice might not be totally objective or worthy of your deference and respect.

6   Feminist Critiques of Obstetrics

Over the last forty years, a robust discussion has taken place about what might be called the philosophy of obstetrics. In oversimplified terms, it has been a debate between the medical profession, or at least the obstetricians, and feminist critics of the modern obstetrical approach to pregnancy and childbirth.

Many of the feminist critics suggest that modern obstetrics fundamentally misunderstands the spiritual as well as the physiological essence of pregnancy and childbirth. By this view, modern obstetrics is committed to the view that pregnancy, labor, and delivery are not natural and healthy events in the lives of women but, instead, are medical problems akin to a disease. The medical profession, by contrast, sees pregnancy as a risky and even potentially life-threatening event that can be made much safer by judicious monitoring and, when necessary, medical interventions. The two different views of pregnancy lead to two very different sorts of ideas about how best to care for and assist the pregnant woman, both during pregnancy and during labor and delivery. The critics of medicalization claim that many of the medical and surgical treatments that obstetricians routinely offer, or even insist upon, are not just unnecessary. They are both medically and psychologically harmful. They represent a fundamental misunderstanding of the naturalness of pregnancy, labor, and delivery. The misunderstanding has dire consequences, not just for pregnancy itself but also for the way we view women's place in the world. To understand the naturalness of pregnancy is to understand the unique power that women have. The medical view makes women weak and dependent. The feminist view allows women to tap into the power of their unique, life-giving capacities. Properly understood, then, pregnancy can empower women. Improperly understood in the ways that today's doctors misunderstand, obstetrics disempowers them.

One of the first books to make this argument was Suzanne Arms's 1977 *Immaculate Deception.* Arms wrote about her own experiences giving birth and about her research into alternatives to the typical hospital birth.[1]

She wrote that "We must question the medical community's insistence that laboring women give birth in the doctor's institution." Her book described how, in hospitals, women in childbirth were routinely separated from their partners, physically restrained at the wrists and ankles, lowered into the stirruped lithotomy position, administered drugs without their consent, given episiotomies without their consent, discouraged from breastfeeding, and not allowed to breastfeed, hold, or even see their babies following delivery.[2]

The book criticized virtually every aspect of obstetrics. Arms wrote, "What is legitimately criticized as obstetrical interference on the outside is promoted as 'medical improvement' on the inside; what is historically considered the sole responsibility of birthing women on the outside is reduced to a matter of 'doctor's orders' or 'hospital policy' on the inside; and what are correctly defined as deceptions on the outside are generally acknowledged as 'scientific fact' on the inside" (p. 52). She criticized efforts to induce labor: "Induced labor so often alters the process from its natural rhythm that the mother cannot maintain control. She believes her body has gone haywire, and becomes frantic in her effort to keep up with contractions that continuously catch her off guard" (p. 58). She criticized fetal heart monitoring as "a lengthy and difficult procedure...that is unnecessary in normal birth." She characterized the drugs that are given during labor as an attempt to "manipulate the process for the convenience of the doctor and the hospital staff" (p. 66) and described how women are convinced to undergo episiotomies by false claims that the alternative is to have a "ragged tear" of the perineal tissue or by the equally false warning that, without an episiotomy, their husbands will no longer enjoy sexual intercourse. She suggested that the position in which doctors place women during labor and delivery, supine with their legs elevated in stirrups, "is obstructive of the birth process in that it works against natural forces of gravity that are helping the baby to find its way into the birth canal." In that position, women are necessarily "sluggish, inactive, and immobile." The supine position, like so many other aspects of modern obstetrics, is recommended, according to Arms, only for the convenience of the doctor, not because it is the best position to facilitate pushing and delivery. She called the purported benefits of modern obstetrics "one of the greatest deceptions of all." She described the typical medicalized birth as "agonizingly slow, impersonal, inefficient, and risky to both mother and child" (p. 54).

Arms's arguments resonated with many women throughout the world. Her book inspired social scientists like Emily Martin and Barbara Katz Rothman to analyze childbirth from anthropological and sociological perspectives. Martin echoes many of

Arms's critiques in her book *The Woman in the Body: A Cultural Analysis of Reproduction*.[3] In that book Martin reviews the ways in which scientific understandings of women's bodies, and of menstruation, childbirth, and menopause, have been shaped throughout history by sociocultural views about gender. Martin summarizes the tensions thus: "Medical imagery juxtaposes two pictures: the uterus as a machine that produces the baby, and the woman as laborer who produces the baby...What role is the doctor given? I think it is clear that he is predominantly seen as the supervisor or foreman of the labor process."[4] Martin shows how these approaches to obstetrics grow out of the larger sociocultural setting within which the medical approaches took shape. She analyzes the language in standard medical textbooks and shows that these books "reveal two fundamental assumptions about women's bodies. First, they assume that female reproductive organs are organized as if they form a hierarchical, bureaucratic organization under centralized control. Second, they assume that women's bodies are predominantly for the purpose of production of desirable substances, primarily babies."[5] These views lead to an industrialized approach to obstetrical care.

Abby Hyde and Bernadette Roche-Reid interviewed 12 midwives about their experiences. Their research supports many of the themes that were articulated by Arms and Martin. Like Martin, they compared the modern obstetrics ward to a childbirth factory with "reproduction treated as form of production."[6] Women become the raw materials. Obstetricians develop techniques to transform those raw materials into manufactured products.

In this childbirth factory, the techniques of obstetrics are designed to facilitate the economically efficient management of women in labor. Standard, unnecessary, and unnatural techniques to achieve this goal include the artificial rupture of membranes, the pharmacologic stimulation of labor, and the ready use of C-sections if either pregnancy or labor lasts longer than is deemed appropriate. The goal of such an approach, according to these critiques, is not to enhance or protect the health of the woman or the baby but instead to maximize the efficiency of the obstetrical ward.

These writers concluded that modern obstetrics does more harm than good. It leads, they claimed, to many unnecessary and harmful invasive procedures. "The instrumental rationality of obstetrics," they wrote, "is linked to an outcome orientation to power and money, and a political economy perspective of medicine."

The sociologist Barbara Katz Rothman also saw modern labor and delivery suites as factories and the modern management of labor as a form of industrial production that emphasizes the efficient removal of a fetus from a woman's body."[7] This approach "takes birth away from the control of the individual woman and her close, matriarchal support system, and places it in the hands of the patriarchal world of medicine and the institutions (i.e., hospitals) at which this approach to health care is practiced."[8]

These early feminist critiques of obstetrics led to a second generation of critical analysis that is, in some ways, more nuanced. This second wave of feminist critiques examines not only the standard practices of obstetrics but also the experiences of women who are being cared for by the mainstream medical system. Jennifer Block, a former editor of Ms. Magazine and an editor of *Our Bodies, Ourselves*, wrote a book about modern obstetrics entitled *Pushed: The Painful Truth about Childbirth and Modern Maternity Care*. Like Arms, Martin, and Rothman, Block gives detailed critiques of many aspects of modern obstetrics, including electronic fetal monitoring, inductions of labor, most

C-sections, episiotomies, and hospital births. She advocates for women to turn their backs on mainstream obstetrics and to opt, instead, for home childbirth with midwives. She also addresses more contemporary issues such as the risks and benefits of vaginal birth after C-sections and the advisability of vaginal births for twins or babies in the breech position.

On these matters, her own views are quite clear.

Block thinks that modern obstetrical practices are blatantly counterproductive. She writes,

The typical obstetric patient now goes through a battery of tests, screens, and ultrasounds during pregnancy. She meets with genetics counselors and weighs whether to get an amniocentesis. She is put through sensitive glucose challenges and increasingly diagnosed with gestational diabetes, although such diagnoses have not improved outcomes. There is new worry over Group B streptococcus (a bacterium commonly found in the vagina) causing infection in the baby—a 0.01% chance. Though screening for such conditions results in more false-positives than accurate diagnoses—and in unnecessary interventions—all women are tested. (p. 58)

The result of all this testing, in Block's view, is that all pregnancies come to be seen as high risk, more and more pregnancies end in medical interventions, and, as a result, "the value of spontaneous vaginal birth—the conditioning of the fetal lungs, the priming of the breastfeeding relationship, the infusion of the 'love hormone,' the physical proximity of mother and baby—is a radical notion among some obstetric leaders" (p. 142).

While Block's own position is clear, she presents both sides of the issue. In the last chapter, she discusses with some bafflement the ways in which debates about childbirth have led to some very strange bedfellows. She describes a couple, Amber and John Marlowe, who "narrowly escaped a court-ordered cesarean" (p. 269). The Marlowes are deeply religious and anti-abortion. They also believe in home births. As a result of their childbirth experiences, in which they had to fight against the government in order to have a baby the way they wanted to, they joined the pro-choice "March for Women's Lives" in Washington in April 2003. According to Block, "they realized that if the government can restrict a woman's right to abortion, then it can force a woman to have a cesarean." Block also interviews Wendy Chavkin, MD, chair of Physicians for Reproductive Choice and Health. Chavkin was a longtime supporter of the pro-choice movement and an advocate of abortion access. But on the issue of vaginal birth after C-section, she defends policies that allow hospitals to prohibit women who have had a cesarean delivery to have a subsequent vaginal birth. "Like many within the medical field," Block writes, "Chavkin has come to see physiologic childbirth as an inherently dangerous procedure that can be withheld" (p. 269). These discussions show that critiques of obstetrics are not all coming from the left. The usual battle lines of our culture wars do not always hold when it comes to childbirth.

Liza Mundy's book about new reproductive technologies, *Everything Conceivable*, describes a similar set of tensions and confusions.[9] "As I got further into the reporting," she writes,

The dilemmas were more complex, and the people facing them more diverse, than I had anticipated. I interviewed married couples, single mothers, lesbian partners, gay fathers. I interviewed parents of twins, parents of triplets, parents who had twins and triplets both. I interviewed egg donors who had contributed genetic material to make a baby possible for another person. I interviewed surrogates or, as they are called now, 'gestational carriers': women who gestate a child for another person, a child who is sometimes biologically related to the surrogate herself, but often not related to her, biologically, at all.

Mundy, too, ends up recognizing that the issues surrounding new reproductive technologies are ones that don't map easily onto old political dividing lines. She describes the debates among members of the President's Council on Bioethics: "Even like-minded conservatives had trouble reaching consensus." She describes similar debates among attendees at a Planned Parenthood meeting: "There are times when we have to acknowledge that we don't know which team we're on. With most reproductive technologies, I think that most of us are genuinely unsure."

There are so many feminist critiques of obstetrics, written from so many perspectives and taking such varied disciplinary approaches (including history, anthropology, sociology, semiotics, personal narrative, and others), that it is difficult to summarize this line of criticism or to do justice to the subtlety and complexity of the analyses. But there are common themes in most such analyses. They generally conclude that modern obstetrics leads to, allows, and perhaps encourages many medical interventions during pregnancy that are unnecessary, invasive, and expensive. They imagine that women would be better off if they sought a return to a less technological, more natural, more individualized approach to pregnancy and childbirth.

Some critiques posit a self-interested economic motive for the obstetric approach to pregnancy. But many see the driving force as something deeper and more philosophical. They hypothesize that modern obstetrics grows out of a disparaging view of women's cognitive and physical abilities. They see modern childbirth as an instantiation of the view that women are fundamentally incapable of taking care of themselves, with the pregnant woman as the ultimate example of helplessness. Pregnant women need an interventionist obstetrician to improve the natural processes of childbearing and thus improve outcomes for themselves and their children. By this view, doctors are not doing what they do simply to make money. They are doing what they do because their fundamental (mis)beliefs about women lead them inevitably to the medicalized approach to pregnancy labor and delivery. In contrast, the feminist critique of this view posits that women are quite capable of taking care of themselves in every aspect of their lives, including pregnancy. In fact, since pregnancy is the most unique female experience, it is the one where women's empowerment is most crucial.

This line of criticism spreads out from the management of labor and delivery—the end-game, as it were, of pregnancy— to examine the whole panoply of reproductive technologies, including infertility treatments,[10] surrogate mother arrangements,[11] obstetrical ultrasound,[12] amniocentesis, and preimplantation genetic diagnosis,[13] among others.

The blurred battle lines and strange bedfellows arise because two sorts of feminism are at work. One is the view that women are empowered only when they take control of their lives in a very particular way, the natural way. This is as prescriptive, in its own way, as is the obstetrical worldview. That is, in positing that modern obstetrics is harmful and that a more natural approach to childbirth is preferable, this critique of obstetrics also, and paradoxically, claims to know what is best for women. But there is another sort of feminist response to the dilemmas of childbirth, a decidedly nonprescriptive view, that sees women's empowerment as a phenomenon that must not necessarily culminate in one particular approach to pregnancy and childbirth but, instead, must recognize and support the ability of women to choose from an ever-broadening range of choices. By this view, women should be able to choose when and how to conceive a baby, what sort of prenatal care and prenatal testing they want or need, what sort of delivery to have. The broader the range of choices, the greater freedom women will have to control their own lives. Of course, the broader the range of choices, the more decisions women must make and the more anxiety they might feel about making the right choices.

This framework highlights two consistent tensions in the feminist critiques of obstetrics. One tension is between, on the one hand, the dehumanizing and commodifying aspects of modern obstetrics and, on the other hand, the claims that these approaches to childbirth lead to better outcomes. Some amount of "dehumanization" may be acceptable and even desirable if it leads to better outcomes for both mother and baby. By contrast, the dehumanization is doubly objectionable if, in fact, it leads to more health problems.

The other tension is between the perceived paternalism of modern obstetrics and the fact that many women seek out and count on new reproductive technologies and high-tech obstetrics. This raises questions of how women's own autonomous choices ought to be understood by those who may disagree with the choices but strongly defend the individual's right to make those choices.

Two debates illustrate the first tension. One is a debate about home birth. The other is about the benefits or harms of caesarean deliveries. That debate, in turn, leads to a controversy that illustrates the second tension; that is, the debate about whether it is appropriate to do a C-section solely because the pregnant woman prefers that method of delivery to a vaginal childbirth. The next chapter addresses the issues that arise from these debates.

7 The Debate about Home Birth

The debate about home birth is as bitter and intractable as the national debate about the Affordable Care Act. Disagreements about the safety of home birth illustrate the ways that people can look at the same data and come to opposite conclusions, so the debate seems impervious to conclusions based on data. There is a boatload of data from dozens of studies conducted in different settings and different countries. The researchers come to different conclusions about the safety or desirability of home birth. Sometimes, the researchers themselves draw one conclusion and an editorial comment on the study comes to the opposite conclusion.

Professional societies in different countries interpret the data differently and thus take different positions about endorsing or prohibiting home birth. In 2008, the American College of Obstetricians and Gynecologists reiterated its long-standing opposition to home births, writing that "childbirth decisions should not be dictated or influenced by what's fashionable, trendy, or the latest cause célèbre. Despite the rosy picture painted by home birth advocates, a seemingly normal labor and delivery can quickly become life-threatening for both the mother and baby."[1] In their opinion, the choice to deliver at home prioritizes the choice of a style for giving birth over the goal of having a healthy baby. On the other side of the Atlantic, the Royal College of Obstetricians and Gynaecologists in the United Kingdom supports home birth for women with uncomplicated pregnancies.[2] The Royal College states, "There is no reason why home birth should not be offered to women at low risk of complications and it may confer considerable benefits for them and their families."

Part of the reason for the controversy is that conclusions about the advisability of home birth reflect different ideas about which risks and benefits are most important. Researchers also present different ideas about how to lower risk. Before we delve into the issues, we must first present a welter of facts and figures. Then we will summarize the conclusions others have drawn, and offer an interpretation of our own.

There is broad agreement on this: *Most studies of home births among carefully selected, low-risk women find that it is about as safe as hospital birth.* In that sentence, though, there are a lot of fudge words. Disagreement centers on the meaning of terms like "carefully selected" and "low-risk" and "about as safe." In those terms lies the root of the controversy.

Some of the best research on the safety of home births has been done in the Canadian province of British Columbia. There, in 1998, the provincial government decided to legalize home births attended by certified nurse-midwives. As part of the legalization, the government mandated that rigorous studies be carried out on outcomes of home births where practitioners followed strict protocols. Patricia Janssen, an epidemiologist, assembled a multidisciplinary team of clinicians and scientists, including obstetricians, midwives, pediatricians, and statisticians, to conduct those studies.

Janssen and colleagues studied all planned home births in British Columbia between 2000 and 2004.[3] They compared those to two other groups: (1) hospital births that met criteria used in the governmental regulations for classifying women as low risk when those births were attended by the same midwives who attended home births; and (2) births that were matched by demographics and risk factors and were attended by physicians in hospitals. The women in this third group were matched with women in the midwife groups based upon age, parity (first birth versus subsequent births), year of the birth, and marital status. The primary outcome measure was perinatal mortality, including both stillbirth after 20 weeks of gestation and death in the first week of life. The researchers also tallied obstetrical interventions for the pregnant women and medical problems among the newborn babies.

During the five-year study period, more than 12,000 women were enrolled. There were 2,899 in the planned home birth group, 4,752 in the planned hospital birth with midwife group, and 5,331 who planned a doctor-attended hospital birth. There were some differences between the groups. Those who planned a home birth were less likely to be single parents or to be having their first baby.

The researchers found that, in all three groups, perinatal mortality was quite low. The rate was lower than 1 in 1,000 perinatal deaths overall, and no statistically significant differences were found between the mortality rates in the three groups. The low overall mortality suggests that the criteria for classifying births as low-risk were good ones. The researchers did find statistically significant differences in other aspects of labor and delivery. Women who had a physician-attended hospital birth were more likely to have had electronic fetal monitoring, augmentation of labor, and analgesic medications. Rates of vaginal delivery were 90% in the home birth group, 82% in the hospital-midwife group, and 75% for the hospital physician group. The physician-attended group of women had more post-delivery infections. Maternal complications were low in each group. There were no infant deaths in any group between 8 and 28 days of age. Babies who were born in hospital were less likely to be readmitted in the first weeks after discharge than were babies born at home.

The authors conclude, "Our study showed that planned home birth attended by a registered midwife was associated with very low and comparable rates of perinatal death and reduced rates of obstetric interventions and adverse maternal outcomes compared with planned hospital birth attended by a midwife or physician." In other words, home birth with a midwife, for this carefully selected group of low-risk women, is as good for the baby and better for the woman than is hospital birth.

An accompanying editorial questions the validity of these conclusions. "As with most studies of home birth," write McLachlan and Foster, "Their study was limited by the possibility—if not the likelihood—of self-selection by participants to a home-birth option. Any differences in outcomes between the study groups may therefore be attributable to differences in the characteristics of the groups themselves."[4]

Is the glass half empty or half full? Is home birth safe only for the sort of people who might choose home birth? If so, what exactly is it about such women that allows them to be such good judges of their own suitability for home birth? Janssen and colleagues acknowledge these complexities. But they see them as a strength of the study, not a weakness, "We cannot exclude the possibility that differences in findings between the groups were attributable to unmeasured characteristics of the women who chose home birth. This self-selection may be an important component of risk management for home birth and in that context is a desirable facet of study design." In other words, they say, home birth is safe for women who both meet objective criteria for being low risk and who choose to have a home birth. Such women, after all, are the ones who will be most affected by the policy of allowing home births. Nobody is required to have a home birth. The question is whether it is a safe option for the women who choose to do so.

A very similar debate has taken place in Sweden. Health policy regarding home birth in Sweden is more like that in the United States than that in British Columbia. According to a Swedish health department website, "The health authorities do not recommend, and seldom fund, home births. A woman who wishes to give birth at home has to find a licensed midwife willing to assist her and she must also pay for the service herself."[5] Nevertheless, some women seek home births with licensed nurse-midwives. Lindgren and colleagues used a population-based registry, and a diligent effort to identify all births in which women either planned to—or actually did—deliver at home, in order to study the outcomes of planned home births in Sweden under these circumstances. They compared outcomes in these pregnancies to outcomes in 11,000 births randomly selected from the national birth database. They were studying outcomes during the twelve years from 1992 to 2004. They compared women who delivered at home with women from the same geographic regions who delivered in the hospital. They looked only at singleton births.

There were many differences between the women in the planned home birth group and the hospital group. Women in the planned home birth group were more often older than 35 years and born in a European country other than Sweden. They were less likely to be unemployed, less likely to smoke, and less likely to be obese. There was no difference in marital status or pre-pregnancy diseases. So, as in Canada, they were a carefully self-selected group. Unlike in the Canadian study, they were not matched with similar women. Instead, they were compared to all women who had babies in a hospital.

The study found that perinatal mortality was nearly four times as high in the home birth group, where 2 of 897 (0.22%) babies died, compared to rate of 7 in 11,341 (0.06%) in the hospital group. The rates in both groups were very low—lower than in most other countries. Because there were so few deaths in either group, even the fourfold difference was not statistically significant, meaning it could well have happened by chance. The C-section rates and rates of delivery by vacuum extraction were 3 to 4 times higher in the hospital birth group. Women who delivered in the hospital were ten times more likely to have an episiotomy. Because the researchers were looking only at live births, they did not have data on stillbirths.

An accompanying editorial notes, "Women should be aware that in a Scandinavian/Nordic context homebirth cannot provide the same safety as a hospital birth." Rates of home birth in Sweden remain low, and the Swedish health system still does not pay for home births.

Two other large studies tried to determine whether or not home birth was safe. Johnson and Davis studied 5,418 planned, midwife-attended home births in the United States and Canada in the year 2000.[6] They found that 12.1% of the women who planned to deliver at home ended up being transferred to the hospital at some point during labor. The rest delivered at home. Overall rates of obstetrical intervention among the group that planned a home birth were lower than those seen in "low-risk" hospital births. Infant mortality outcomes were no different. They concluded, "Planned home birth for low risk women in North America using certified professional midwives was associated with lower rates of medical intervention but similar intrapartum and neonatal mortality to that of low risk hospital births in the United States."

Pang and colleagues, by contrast, found that, among 5,854 planned home deliveries in Washington State in the years 1989 through 1996, there was an increased risk for neonatal death.[7] "Infants of planned home deliveries were at increased risk of neonatal death and Apgar score no higher than 3 at 5 minutes. These same relationships remained when the analysis was restricted to pregnancies of at least 37 weeks' gestation." These results generated vigorous discussion among readers, most of which made points similar to those made by editorialists about the Canadian and Swedish studies.

The Cochrane Collaborative, an organization that specializes in meta-analyses of data on the safety and efficacy of medical procedures, reviewed the data on the safety of home birth.[8] They noted that most studies of home birth were observational studies, rather than prospective randomized trials. They discuss the problems with such studies and the reasons why those problems make it impossible to draw any firm conclusions. They conclude their analysis with unambiguous uncertainty:

Most pregnancies among healthy women are normal, and most births could take place without unnecessary medical intervention. However, it is not possible to predict with certainty that absolutely no complications will occur in the course of a birth...It seems increasingly clear that impatience and easy access to many medical procedures at hospital may lead to increased levels of intervention which in turn may lead to new interventions and finally to unnecessary complications. In a planned home birth assisted by an experienced midwife with collaborative medical backup in case transfer should be necessary these drawbacks are avoided while the benefit of access to medical intervention when needed is maintained. Increasingly better observational studies suggest that planned hospital birth is not any safer than planned home birth assisted by an experienced midwife with collaborative medical back up, but may lead to more interventions and more complications. However, there is no strong evidence from randomised trials to favour either planned hospital birth or planned home birth for low-risk pregnant women.

But uncertainty, in this context, is actually an endorsement of the permissibility of home birth. If the data cannot show that home birth is more dangerous, then that data would support the idea that women should be able to choose. After all, in most medical situations, when there is no proven difference in efficacy between two treatments, we generally let patients decide which they prefer.

The Dutch Experience

The Netherlands is the only country in Western Europe in which the health system not only tolerates and supports but actually encourages home births. Their system, as the sociologist Raymond De Vries has noted, is "a glaring exception in the world of modern obstetrics."[9] As De Vries describes it:

Measured in terms of health outcomes or by its use of sophisticated technology, the medical system of the Netherlands rivals that of any nation, and yet nearly one-third of the births there take place at home.

This number stands in stark contrast to the rest of the developed world: in no other country with a modern health system do more than 3% of births occur at home. Midwives are primary attendants at 71% of Dutch home births; they attend 48% of all of that nation's births. It is a system that works quite well in terms of cost-efficiency and quality. The high midwife attended home birth rate is coupled with the world's lowest rates of surgical intervention in birth and very low rates of infant mortality.[10]

For many years, the example of the Dutch system was used as a trump card in arguments about the safety of home birth. If the Dutch could do it, then everybody could do it. And if everybody did it, proponents argued, then all pregnant women would get better care during labor and delivery with fewer of the complications associated with hospital-based obstetrics, they would have excellent perinatal care outcomes, and overall cost would be much lower.

That argument and conclusion are not as straightforward as they seem. The success of the Dutch system may not be so easily replicated in other countries. Because of the long tradition of midwifery in The Netherlands, the Dutch have a highly developed system for training midwives. Midwives there are trained in unique, rigorous, five-year midwifery academies. In order to replicate the Dutch experience, other countries would have to create a whole new system of training for midwives.

The Dutch themselves are not so sure that would be such a good idea. They have debated the pros and cons of their approach for fifty years and have made adjustments in their system along the way. In the 1960s, two-thirds of births in the Netherlands took place at home. In recent years, the percentage of home births has dropped to about one-third. This is still higher than in any other industrialized country, but the rate is steadily falling. The reasons for the change are important.

There is considerable debate, within and outside the Netherlands, about both the reasons for the uniqueness of the Dutch and about the consequences of their system. In 2009, van Weel and colleagues summarized the debate.[11] They noted that most discussions about the safety or desirability of home birth intermingle three different sets of concerns. The first is the quality of the evidence about the effect of the place of birth (home or

hospital) on outcomes. The second, related issue is the effectiveness of risk selection in primary midwifery care. How good are
midwives at figuring out which women truly are low risk? The
third issue is the question of whether women in the Netherlands
make truly informed choice. Until recently, the Dutch insurance system did not pay for hospital birth for women who were
deemed by midwives to be low risk.

The second issue forms the basis for the third. As van Weel et
al. note, "Timely and appropriate obstetric risk selection is deli-
cate. Adverse events may occur if too few or too many women are
referred, or referrals are made too early or too late. If women are
not referred in time, perinatal outcomes may be worse in primary
midwife-led care compared with those in obstetrician-led care.
On the other hand, unnecessary referrals may increase the risk
of unnecessary obstetric interventions...The quality of risk assessment is vital in this context, in this case to help the pregnant
woman to make an informed choice for her place of delivery."

The Dutch experience is also unique and complicated because
the Dutch health care system is also unique. It offers citizens different types of health insurance coverage. The wealthiest third of
the population purchase private insurance without any government assistance. Some in this group receive help from employers
in paying premiums while others pay the whole bill themselves.
The other two-thirds of the Dutch population is covered under
a compulsory state-run health insurance scheme financed by
deductions from wages. Under this system, the government has
an incentive to keep costs down. One of the ways it does so is
by incentivizing the use of midwives and home deliveries. How
does this work? De Vries describes the system:

The government believes that unlimited choice for childbearing women
could spell the end of midwife-assisted home birth, thus raising costs

and harming the quality of birth care. For this reason Dutch women whose pregnancies proceed "normally" are not free to choose specialist care: these women must use primary care and can be attended either at home or in a polyclinic. This injunction is maintained via the insurance system (women with "normal" pregnancies and births will not be reimbursed for specialist care) and by professional custom (specialists will not attend normal births.)[12]

In the last few years, the Dutch system has changed. A health reform law was passed in 2006. The government no longer incentivizes home birth. Perhaps as a result, the number of women delivering at home has declined in the last few years. (It had declined rapidly in the 1970s, but then had held steady for a few decades.)

How are the outcomes in the Netherlands? Not surprisingly, there is some controversy. A collaborative study of perinatal mortality in 26 European countries showed that the Netherlands had the highest rates of both fetal death and neonatal death among all the countries in the study.[13] Careful analysis revealed a number of contributing factors, but left open questions about the contribution of home births. The authors of this comparative study of different European countries cautiously concluded that "perinatal health and the quality of perinatal healthcare deserve a more prominent position in Dutch research programmes." An accompanying editorial argued that this result had nothing to do with the Dutch system of home deliveries. Instead, Merkus argued, "It is more likely that the attitude of Dutch professionals is too expectative, based on too much confidence in a non-intervention policy." By this, he seemed to be referring to two things. First, at the time of the study, the Dutch had not used prenatal screening as commonly as did other countries. Thus, they were less likely to make prenatal diagnoses of congenital anomalies and had lower rates of abortion for such congenital anomalies. This lead, in turn, to higher rates of neonatal mortality associated with those anomalies. Dutch neonatologists were also relatively noninterventionist, compared to the rest of Europe, for babies born at the borderline of viability. Thus, their infant mortality rates for tiny premature babies were higher than in other countries. Merkus called for better prenatal screening and the introduction of preconception care rather than a shift away from home birth.[14] He might also have suggested that infant mortality rates be adjusted to take into account the effect of policies regarding treatment for babies born at the borderline of viability.

It is clear from the ongoing debate about the Dutch system of perinatal care, both within Holland and outside of it, that the Dutch data will not resolve the question of whether home birth is safer, as safe, or riskier than hospital delivery. Instead, the Dutch data simply reinforce the conclusion that one reaches after analyzing debates in other countries and other places: home birth is very safe for some women under some circumstances, but the decision about where to have a baby remains complex for both pregnant women and the professionals who attend to them during childbirth.

Furthermore, home birth must be evaluated in the context of the overall health care system. In the Netherlands, the tradition of midwifery no doubt results in a cadre of midwives with different skills and experiences than midwives in other countries. Such differences in culture and in national health policies shape the ways in which obstetrical interventions can be evaluated. Because of the normality of home birth in the Netherlands, the factors associated with women having a home birth are different there than in other countries, making it hard to generalize from the Dutch experience. In other countries the essential determinant of home birth is the personal ideology of the mother. Women only have births at home if they choose to do so. Once women make that decision, they need to find a professional who will attend their home birth. In the Netherlands, by contrast, the clinical judgment of an experienced midwife is the primary determinant of the place of birth for most women. The only way that selection factors could ever be ruled out as overriding determinants of outcomes observed for home versus hospital deliveries would be if women were randomly assigned to receive one or the other. But a study allowing that decision to be made by chance is one few women would be likely to participate in.

While the debate about home birth is interesting and reveals a major fault line in perinatal policy and philosophy, it is not so relevant to a woman like you. You thought about home birth. You decided against it. You opted for a low-tech birthing center birth. That plan is not working out so well. Now, you have to decide whether to authorize a C-section. A preterm C-section. You understand the reasons why you perhaps should trust your doctor. You understand the caveats. But how bad would it really be to have a C-section? Why not just have the operation, get the baby out, and get on with your life?

There is a debate within obstetrics about how bad—or how good—C-sections might be. This debate has gotten less publicity than the one about home birth. But there are a lot more C-sections than there are home births. Maybe studies should be done to more carefully examine the risks and, yes, benefits of C-sections. Some doctors believe that more C-sections might be good both for women and for their babies.

8 Are C-sections Good for Women (and Babies, Too)?

So what if you decide to have a C-section? You don't want an operation. You want to do what is best for your baby. If you needed an operation, you'd have one, but do you need one? How dangerous would a C-section be for you, either in the short term or over the long haul? Of all the controversies swirling around obstetrics today, one of the weirdest ones is a controversy about whether women should be permitted to request a C-section even when there are no medical indications. It is a controversy that illustrates some of the difficulties in assessing the risks and benefits of this operation. It also highlights fissures in feminist philosophy. As noted above, one stream of feminist thought suggests that women need to be empowered to resist the medicalization of pregnancy and to insist on natural childbirth. Another stream suggests that empowerment must allow women to make their own choices and to decide when and how they want to have their babies. The latter view turns the argument about physician-induced demand on its head. Maybe the rising rate of C-sections is not a consequence of doctors trying to maximize their own income and well-being by convincing women to do something that the women do not want to do but, instead, reflects women's own preferences for a certain type of delivery or a certain risk-benefit trade-off. Evidence for this contrarian interpretation of the driving forces behind C-section trends comes from the observation that many obstetricians refuse to do C-sections if there is no medical indication to do one. They do this even though they could make more money by doing more C-sections and even though some of their patients are requesting that the C-sections be done in these circumstances.

In 2006, the National Institutes of Health convened a consensus conference to examine the phenomenon labeled "C-section on maternal demand" or CSMD.[1] The participants acknowledged that there is no good data on how common CSMD is or even how, exactly, to define it. Many C-sections take place after a discussion between a pregnant woman and her doctor in which the risks and benefits of C-section, compared to vaginal delivery, are discussed and evaluated. In some of these situations, the doctor may recommend a C-section. In others, the woman may request it. The subtleties of those conversations and the process of shared decision making both lead to ambiguity in the classification of any particular C-section as one undertaken following a "maternal demand."

Although the general criteria for classifying C-sections as CSMDs are not well defined, for a particular subset of C-sections there is little ambiguity. In that subset, there is no bona fide medical indication and the doctor and the pregnant woman each agree that the reason for the C-section is the woman's preferred mode and timing of delivery.

The NIH consensus conference examined all available evidence regarding the frequency with which such procedures were done, and reviewed the outcome data for the procedure. The report begins by acknowledging the difficulty in determining how frequently such procedures are performed. They cite studies, but most are anecdotal, single-center, and methodologically inadequate. The best data come not from the United States but from a survey of obstetricians in Australia that showed that, in 2006, there were 8,553 maternal-request cesarean deliveries. This represented 17% to 25% of all pre-labor C-sections, and 3.2% to 4.7% percent of all births in Australia.[2]

Regardless of exactly how common or uncommon CSMDs are, they illustrate an important debate in the ethics of obstetrics. The guiding ethical principles of obstetrics can prioritize either the woman's autonomy or the doctor's obligation to do no harm. Autonomy-based arguments claim that women should have the right to determine whether to have a C-section or a vaginal birth. By such arguments, women's freedom should be limited only if they are requesting something that is known to be harmful. Then, doctors may have a competing claim of professional autonomy that empowers them to refuse to cause harm to a patient without any compensatory benefit. Thus, C-sections without medical indications, done following the request of a pregnant woman, can be ethically acceptable only if the procedure is thought to be safe for both the woman and her baby. The resolution of the debate, then, turns on whether the risks of C-sections are outweighed by the benefits.

In 2006, the same year as the NIH consensus conference, Bettes and colleagues surveyed 1,031 members of the American College of Obstetrics and Gynecology regarding their opinions about doing C-sections based on the patient's request without a medical indication. The obstetricians were evenly divided. About half objected and said that they would refuse to do a C-section under those circumstances. Half believed that women have the right to request and receive a cesarean delivery and stated that they would be willing to perform one. Many of the survey respondents reported that they had, in fact, done such C-sections in the past.[3] Doctors who acceded to patient requests for medically nonindicated C-sections were more likely to see benefits from the procedure and less likely to see risks.

The risks are clear. A C-section is a surgical operation and can cause maternal morbidity and mortality. Some studies show higher neonatal mortality rates. But even critics of C-sections acknowledge that mortality for either mother or baby is very rare. All acknowledge that C-sections can have long-term detrimental consequences, such as an increase in the risk of uterine hemorrhage during later pregnancies. Even that risk, though, has become less important in an era when women have fewer pregnancies and fewer babies.

Not all C-sections are alike in terms of risk. Elective C-sections are safer than ones done in emergency situations. Emergency C-sections are more likely to occur if doctors and their patients choose not to do them electively. In that situation, if they attempt to deliver the baby vaginally and things do not go well, they may have to operate emergently.

Vaginal deliveries, while generally safer, do increase the risk of certain complications. Women who deliver vaginally are more likely to have long-term problems with urinary incontinence than women who have a C-section. Injuries to the anal sphincter are also more common after vaginal delivery.[4,5]

So how do the experts balance these risks for themselves? Wu and colleagues surveyed members of the American Urogynecologic Society (AUGS) and members of the Society for Maternal-Fetal Medicine (SMFM) about their attitudes regarding C-sections for themselves or their loved ones. The results suggested a difference of opinion between the doctors who focus on the well-being of both mother and baby compared to the doctors who provide care only to women. More than 45% of AUGS respondents stated that they would choose a cesarean delivery for themselves or their partner for their first pregnancy. Among SMFM members, only 9.5% would make the same choice. In a statistical model accounting for each physician's age, sex, years in practice, subspecialty, and whether or not the physician had children, AUGS members were 3.5 times more likely than SMFM members to agree to perform an elective C-section if a woman wanted one.[6] Among members of the Society for Maternal-Fetal Medicine, the two most important considerations in deciding when, if ever, to accede to a request for a C-section were the safety of the procedure and the health of the baby.

Assessments of whether C-sections can lead to better outcomes for the baby are even more complicated than assessments about the risks and benefits to the pregnant woman.

The complication arises, in part, because the risks and benefits for the baby depend upon when and why the C-section is done. If it is done preterm, then the baby is at risk for all of the neonatal complications described above. But most of those complications are not the result of having been born by C-section. They are the result of having been born preterm. To assess the effects on babies that can be attributed to the C-sections themselves, we must examine the consequences of doing C-sections electively at term.

Hankins and colleagues analyzed the likely effects of doing C-section on request at 39 weeks of gestation when there were no other medical indications. They looked at four specific outcomes—shoulder dystocia, fetal trauma, neonatal encephalopathy, and fetal demise.[7]

With regard to neonatal encephalopathy (that is, brain damage caused by lack of oxygen to the brain), their analysis shows that infants born to non-laboring women delivered by C-section had an 83% reduction in the occurrence of moderate or severe encephalopathy. Considering a prevalence of moderate or severe neonatal encephalopathy of 0.38% and applying it to the 3 million deliveries occurring at or after 39 weeks gestational age in the United States annually, they calculated that there are approximately 11,400 cases of moderate to severe encephalopathy annually. If every pregnant woman in the United States had an elective C-section at 39 weeks, the rate of encephalopathy could be cut by nearly 80%. By this calculation, elective C-sections at 39 weeks could prevent nearly 10,000 cases of brain damage annually in the United States.

The potential reduction in fetal demise is equally striking. Copper reported that the rate of stillbirth is constant from 23 to 40 weeks of gestation, with about 5% of all stillbirths occurring at each week of gestation.[8] Yudkin and colleagues noted a rapid rise in the frequency of fetal demise after 39 weeks of gestation, from 0.6 stillbirths per 1,000 live births from 33 to 39 weeks to 1.9 per 1,000 live births at 40 weeks.[9] Hankins and colleagues estimated that induced delivery at 39 weeks would prevent 2 fetal deaths per 1,000 living fetuses. This would translate into the prevention of as many as 6,000 intrauterine fetal deaths in the United States annually.

By these calculations, the benefits of higher rates of C-sections might outweigh the risks. Importantly, the benefits would primarily accrue to the babies while the risks would have a bigger impact on their mothers. This differential allocation of risk highlights the ways in which the nature of both prenatal care and obstetrical care has changed, discussed earlier in the book. Sometimes—perhaps more and more often—prenatal care and obstetrical care focus on the interests of the baby even when those conflict with the interests of the mother. This is a new phenomenon.

The tension between what is good for you as a pregnant woman and what is best for your baby is one that you inevitably must consider as you lie awake at night, trying to decide whether to ask your doctor to intervene and induce an early delivery or whether, instead, you should trust in nature. Life was simpler—though outcomes were worse—when it was impossible to monitor the fetus and the only focus of medical attention was on the health of the pregnant woman. Today, the health of the fetus sometimes takes precedence. We have become much better at monitoring the fetus, and at treating the fetus like a patient.

At the risk of leaving you there, unable to sleep, unable to make a decision, confused by too much data and too few unambiguous conclusions, we are going to shift our focus for a bit and look at the process by which the fetus became a patient. We will do this by recounting some key historical developments that led to the ability to treat a fetus in the womb as a separate patient, discoveries that led to the sort of situation in which you find yourself today. We will come back to you in a few chapters.

9 The Fetus Becomes a Patient

Prenatal care has been fundamentally transformed by our ability to assess the health and the well-being of the fetus independently of the health and well-being of the pregnant woman. That transformation was catalyzed in the middle of the twentieth century by research on two particular conditions—erythroblastosis fetalis (EBF) and Down syndrome (DS).

EBF can now be prevented so it is rarely seen today in developed countries. In the 1940s, however, it was a common cause of both stillbirth and infant mortality. EBF is caused by a mismatch between the blood types of a pregnant woman and her fetus. It used to affect one of every 200 newborns. Furthermore, it ran in families, so afflicted couples would often lose one baby after another.

Down syndrome is caused by a duplication of chromosome 21. The likelihood that a baby will have Down syndrome increases with increasing maternal (and, to a lesser degree, paternal) age. Down syndrome is still very much with us today. The medical techniques that were invented to prenatally diagnose and treat EBF eventually played a major role in the prenatal diagnosis of DS. The two stories are thus intertwined in fascinating ways. Because the stories of these diseases are central to the transformation of prenatal care, we recount them in some detail. The development of techniques to diagnose these conditions allowed the fetus to become a patient.

A. W. Liley and the Treatment of Erythroblastosis Fetalis

In the early twentieth century, Landsteiner identified the existence of the A, B, and O blood groups. Each blood type was characterized by unique substances found on the surfaces of red blood cells. The discovery of blood types allowed safe blood transfusions. Before that, transfusions were often associated with catastrophic and life-threatening reactions. With the discovery of blood types, it became clear that people with the same blood type could safely donate blood to—or receive a donation from—each other but that people reacted badly when transfused with mismatched blood. Sometimes, pregnant women and their fetuses have different blood types and the reactions that occur can be similar to those that occur during blood transfusions.

In 1937, scientists discovered another blood type factor. There is still dispute over who discovered it. (There is a similar debate, as we shall see, about who discovered the presence of an extra chromosome in Down syndrome.) Philip Levine and Alexander Weiner both claim credit for the discovery of Rh factor. The debate became so contentious that the Welcome Trust Center in London held a "witness seminar" in 2003 to try to sort out the competing claims:

Wiener said that he and Landsteiner discovered the Rh factor in humans while they were looking for antisera to as yet undetected blood group factors, and they were doing this by injecting rhesus monkey blood into rabbits and guinea pigs. They named the new antigen, thus revealed, as the rhesus, or Rh antigen. When the antiserum to Rh was tested against human blood, they found that 85 per cent of their samples were Rh positive, 15 per cent were Rh negative. They delayed publication, they claimed, to improve the process of production of the anti-rhesus serum. Their work was not published until 1940, three years after their initial studies, when it became clear that it could explain unexpected haemolytic reactions that arose during blood transfusions between otherwise ABO-identical individuals.[1]

For his part, Levine thought he had priority. In 1937 he had found a previously unknown antiserum in a woman who had given birth to a stillborn infant. This antiserum reacted with the father's red blood cells, but not the mother's. The same antiserum also reacted with 80 per cent of other blood samples with which it was tested. Levine's publication on this case, co-authored with Rufus Stetson, didn't appear until 1939, two years later, but still before Weiner's paper was published.[2]

What is not disputed is that Wiener gave the new factor its name, Rh, and that Levine explained its role in the disease affecting the family whose blood he had studied in 1937.

Levine's discovery that the Rh factor was the cause of EBF allowed the possibility of testing pregnant women for Rh factor. If they were positive, their pregnancies were at risk for the disease. By 1943, such antenatal testing became routine in England. (This was possible, in part, because during World War II in England, laboratories had been set up to do population testing of the blood groups in order to improve the success rates of transfusions to wounded soldiers. The technology was then applied to the care of pregnant women.) This allowed the identification of babies who were at risk for Rh-induced disease. Many fetuses were so severely affected that they did not survive until birth. There was little that could be done in those cases. In other cases, though, babies were less severely affected and survived until birth. The treatment for such babies was to give affected newborns emergency transfusions of Rh-negative blood. There were no neonatal intensive care units and no intravenous catheters small enough for newborns, so these transfusions were usually given intraosseously—directly into the bone marrow—rather than intravenously.

In 1950, Bevis pushed the management of EBF to the next level. He and his colleagues developed a technique to remove a sample of amniotic fluid (or "liquor amnii," as they called it) and to test it for the presence of bilirubin. A higher level of bilirubin indicated more severe disease and could be used to predict which fetuses would die in utero and which would survive until delivery.[3] This was the first time an invasive medical test was used to assess disease in the fetus.

The only intervention that was possible at the time was to induce premature delivery. This was before the development of mechanical ventilation for premature babies, so premature birth was associated with very high mortality rates. Physicians had to weigh the risks of progressive Rh-disease in the fetus against the risks of early delivery. Some fetuses were discovered to be so severely affected at such an early stage of gestation that nothing could be done except to wait for them to die. For others, early delivery seemed to be life-saving. EBF was one of the first examples of prenatal care being used to diagnose a fetal disease for which the treatment was a medically induced preterm delivery. It would be a harbinger of things to come.

In 1963, Liley pioneered a radical advance in the treatment of EBF. He used Bevis's technique of amniocentesis to determine which fetuses were at high risk of intrauterine death. He hypothesized that babies whose amniocentesis results were so dire that death was inevitable could be given an intrauterine blood transfusion that, if successful, would enable them to survive for a few more days or weeks in the womb. Because there was no way to easily visualize the fetus, and no tiny catheters available for transfusions, he proposed to inject the blood not into a vein or even the bone marrow (as would be done for a newborn in those days) but instead to inject it directly into the abdominal cavity of the fetus.

His first case report—the first-ever case report of the treatment of a fetus in the womb—reads almost like science fiction. After describing how, at Bevis's center and others, amniocentesis and early induction of labor had reduced mortality from 22% to 9%, he suggests that it could be reduced further if treatment could be provided to the most severely affected fetuses. He writes, "Transfusion in utero appeared the logical procedure for these very severely affected babies early in the third trimester, and intraperitoneal transfusion seemed the simplest technique."[4]

His first patient was a woman whose fourth pregnancy was in trouble. The woman had previously given birth to one healthy baby but two subsequent pregnancies resulted in intrauterine fetal deaths. An amniocentesis at 30 weeks gestation in the fourth pregnancy showed high levels of bilirubin in the amniotic fluid, a sign of a hopeless prognosis for the infant to survive to term. Liley noted, "The patient and her husband were an intelligent couple, and the prognosis for the foetus, the possibility and uncertainty of intrauterine transfusion, and the potential hazards to the mother were fully explained to and discussed with them." They agreed to try his innovative procedure.

At 32 weeks of gestation, after getting x-rays to determine the position of the fetus, and after sedating the mother, Liley and colleagues conducted the very first intrauterine blood transfusion.

Under local anaesthesia an 8-cm. gauge-16 Tuohy needle was inserted to the amniotic cavity and the stylet withdrawn. A syringe of sterile saline was attached and the needle advanced until resistance to slow steady injection showed that the tip lay in the foetal abdominal wall. With a slight advance free injection was again possible into the foetal peritoneum. No ascitic fluid could be aspirated.

A "portex" epidural catheter shortened to 30 cm. was now fed up to the hub of the Tuohy needle and the needle withdrawn on to the mother's skin. The position of the catheter was checked by x-ray examination and 100 ml. of packed warmed group 0, Rh-negative cells fully compatible with mother's serum was injected over 20 minutes. Antibiotic cover was provided by 1 gram of streptomycin and 1,000,000 units of penicillin injected into the amniotic cavity at amniography, half this dose injected slowly as the catheter was withdrawn through the foetal and maternal tissues, and a four-day course of penicillin and streptomycin given to the mother.

Eight days later an attempt to repeat the transfusion failed. ... However, two days later—that is, at 33 weeks 4 days by dates—a successful puncture was made easily with an 18-cm. gauge-16 Tuohy needle.

At 34 weeks 3 days...a male infant weighing 2,560 g. was delivered. He was pale and slightly jaundiced. The abdomen was moderately distended, with a liver edge palpable 5 cm. below the right costal margin and an easily felt enlarged spleen. Two small pigmented scars in the left lower quadrant of the abdomen showed the puncture sites of the successful transfusions and four smaller scars the pricks of the unsuccessful attempts.

This story is remarkable for a number of reasons. First, it raises interesting questions of research ethics. Liley acknowledged that there is no way to know with certainty that the fetus would have died without treatment. He thus admits that he was doing a potentially risky procedure that could have killed the fetus. This sort of uncertainty often plagues clinical innovation. To the extent that an intervention has risks, it should be used only if the potential benefits outweigh the risks. But the only way to know whether the procedure is beneficial is to try it, in all its riskiness, and to study it to see if it works. Doctors and patients must decide whether the potential risks—all things considered—seem to be lower than the potential benefits. Only careful research can determine whether such gambles pay off.

These problems were recognized in Liley's time as they are today. The editors of the *British Medical Journal* wrote an editorial to accompany Liley's original care report in which they noted, "The procedures involved, however, bear so many hazards to mother and foetus that they can clearly have only a limited application."[5] They saw Liley's technique as a stopgap measure while awaiting a more permanent and safer solution. "The search continues for a method of neutralizing the antibodies in the mother's blood, which would be the most logical way of preventing the disease." That search would eventually culminate in the development of an immunoglobulin that targeted the Rh-positive red blood cell. That immunoglobulin is now routinely given to Rh-negative women at the time of delivery. It prevents them from developing antibodies against Rh-positive red blood cells and so prevents EBF in subsequent pregnancies. It has virtually eliminated EBF in the developed world.

Liley's work opened up a whole new domain of clinical possibilities. It allowed doctors to think about other clinical situations in which fetal diseases could be diagnosed and fetal interventions tried. Liley laid the conceptual foundation for the development of fetal surgery. That field has struggled for decades with the same sort of dilemmas that Liley faced.[6]

Perhaps more important, the work of Liley and Bevis set the stage for a new approach to obstetrics in which the fetus becomes a patient and the goal of prenatal care is not simply to keep the pregnant woman as healthy as possible but also to assess the health and well-being of the fetus in order to make more informed choices about the optimum timing and mode of delivery. Liley, and Bevis before him, explicitly addressed the balance of risks and benefits in continuing a high-risk pregnancy versus inducing an early delivery. The calculus for such decisions would change dramatically once new techniques of caring for premature babies were developed. But even today, the questions that are asked and the calculations that are carried out look very similar to those Liley weighed fifty years ago. This was a new type of prenatal care.

Jerome Lejeune and the Prenatal Diagnosis of Down Syndrome

A second important discovery that changed the nature of prenatal care was reported in August 1958, when Jerome Lejeune, a French cytogeneticist, presented a paper at the International Conference of Genetics in Montreal describing a patient with Down syndrome. Lejeune reported that the baby had a supplementary chromosome, an extra chromosome 21, and that this was the likely cause of the DS. The paper was greeted with interest but also with some skepticism. Most scientists at the time believed that Down syndrome and other congenital anomalies would be explained by single-gene mutations rather than extra chromosomes.

Lejeune and colleagues continued their investigations. In January 1959 they published a paper reporting three children with DS who had the same extra chromosome.[7] A few months later, they followed up this publication with another paper reporting nine children with the same chromosomal anomaly.[8] This paper "confirmed the existence of the first chromosomal aberration in a disease and inaugurated a new discipline: human cytogenetics."[9] The findings were soon confirmed by Jacobs and colleagues.[10]

The discovery that DS was caused by (or at least associated with) an extra chromosome opened up the possibility that, using amniocentesis, the condition could be diagnosed prenatally. This idea was taken up by Steele and Breg, who were at the time using Liley's technique of amniocentesis to diagnose hemolytic disease. They realized that the amniotic fluid they were analyzing for bilirubin levels also contained cells from the fetus. They figured out how to grow those cells in a tissue culture and then to examine the chromosomes within the cells. They published a paper in 1966 describing the results of this technique in 21 patients. They concluded: "A reliable technique for culturing foetal amniotic-fluid cells would...allow more practical genetic counseling of mothers with high risks of having children with chromosomal abnormalities or inborn error of metabolism. Combined with the judicious use of therapeutic abortion, this technique could help reduce the incidence of human chromosomal abnormalities."[11]

This was the first time in medical history that diagnostic tests were done on the fetus in order to determine whether or not to end the pregnancy by an induced abortion. It led to a rapid expansion in the number of centers offering amniocentesis for prenatal diagnosis and, eventually, to refinements of the technique. In 1968, Nadler reported the use of amniocentesis to diagnose a number of cytogenetic and biochemical disorders, including Down syndrome, Hunter syndrome, Pompe's disease, and galactose-1-phosphate uridyltransferase deficiency. At the time of his publication, abortion was illegal in most parts of the United States (In 1967, Colorado, Oregon, California, and North Carolina had passed laws legalizing abortion in certain circumstances.) Nevertheless, Nadler concluded, "Despite the moral, legal, and ethical questions which must be dealt with when therapeutic abortion or modification of genetic traits is considered, attempts at prenatal detection and management are warranted if we are to significantly modify the natural history of these disorders."[12]

Nadler's ideas were picked up on by many others. By 1970, there were ten centers offering prenatal diagnosis through amniocentesis in the United States, and they were increasingly busy. In 1972, Epstein and colleagues wrote, "Diagnostic amniocentesis for the prenatal detection of genetic defects has rapidly established itself as a powerful tool for genetic counseling."[13] By the end of the decade, there were 125 centers in the United States offering amniocentesis.

Lejeune himself was not happy about these developments. He was a devout Catholic and profoundly opposed to abortion. He is surely one of very few individuals ever considered a possible candidate both for a Nobel Prize and for canonization by the Catholic Church. (Mother Teresa achieved both these distinctions, but she won the Nobel Peace Prize, rather than a prize in science.)

He was deeply troubled that his discovery led to the widespread use of prenatal diagnosis and abortion. He had hoped, instead, that his discovery would be used to find a treatment or cure for Down syndrome or, if not, to improve the lives of people with genetic diseases. He went on to create a foundation to foster this work, the Jerome Lejeune Foundation. The mission of the foundation is to support "medical research into intelligence diseases and genetic diseases," and to support the "care and treatment of patients, in particular those suffering from Trisomy 21 or other genetic anomalies, whose lives and dignity must be protected from the moment of conception until they die."[14]

In 1969, Lejeune was awarded the William Allen Memorial Award by the American Society of Human Genetics. This award, the highest honor that the society gives, is presented annually "to recognize substantial and far-reaching scientific contributions to human genetics."[15] It was given to Lejeune in honor of his 1959 paper. As recipient of the award, he was invited to give a speech at the annual meeting of the American Society of Human Genetics in San Francisco.

Lejeune's 1969 Allen lecture was an extended, satiric critique of the whole enterprise of prenatal diagnosis and selective abortion. He entitled his lecture "On the Nature of Men." He chose as an epigraph the following line: "To kill or not to kill, that is the question."[16]

He spoke of his concern, as a geneticist, for "those unfortunate children who do not share equitably our chromosomal heritage," and asked, pointedly, "Should these variants of the human condition be allowed to live?" He proposed that "the answer must be based upon scientific grounds and be as free as possible from emotional or opportunistic reactions." Up to this point, the assembled geneticists were probably with him. They didn't know what was in store.

In order to achieve such scientific rationality, Lejeune suggested that a new scientific institute be created. He called it the National Institute of Death. The new NID, he speculated, would have a fivefold mission:

A. Decree on undesirable genes or chromosomes.
B. Deliver unhappy parents from unwanted pregnancies.
C. Discard embryos not fitting standard requirements.
D. Dispose of newborns not reaching minimal specifications of normalcy.
E. Destroy, delete, or decry any human condition voted against by the NID board of advisors.

To insure that the Board of Advisors of his imagined NID be "objective, rational, scientific, and non-superstitious," he stipulated that "advisors shall be chosen from among knowledgeable persons not belonging to any philosophy, society, or race." Only such people, that is, people with no beliefs, values, or human culture, he bitterly asserted, have the qualifications to determine which pregnancies should be allowed to continue and which should be terminated.

The need for such an Institute, Lejeune suggested, is clear:

Many precise but very complex questions must be solved. For example: is the Turnerian way of life to be accepted? Is the 21-trisomic way of life to be protected?..., and the like. Willy-nilly we come to the conclusion that such a difficult matter, that of deciding what is desirable and should be respected and what is undesirable and should be rejected, deals with considerable "technical" intricacies. In such situations the common practice is not to leave the decision to unprepared or to directly involved persons, but to resort to some jurisdiction, or some body of counselors.

He then spent some time discussing the intricacies of predicting survival, quality of life, or the implications of the survival or eradication of certain genotypes and phenotypes from the human race. He concluded the talk with the following exhortation:

We human geneticists have to face everyday reality: disabled children and distressed parents exist. Should we capitulate in the face of our own ignorance and propose to eliminate those we cannot help? For millennia, medicine has striven to fight for life and health and against disease and death. Any reversal of the order of these terms of reference would entirely change medicine itself. It happens that nature does condemn. Our duty has always been not to inflict the sentence but to try to commute the pain. In any foreseeable genetical trial, I do not know enough to judge, but I feel enough to advocate.

There is no record of how the gathered geneticists reacted to this speech. Lejeune's perspective does, however, crystallize the philosophical tension inherent in fetal medicine. Better techniques for prenatal diagnosis allow us to identify many types of congenital anomalies in the fetus. There is no treatment for most of these anomalies. Instead, the identification of such anomalies allows pregnant women and their doctors to decide whether to terminate the pregnancy.

Lejeune realized just how unpopular his views were among the geneticists. After the speech, he wrote to his wife and said, "Today, I lost my Nobel Prize in medicine."[17]

Did Lejeune Really Discover Trisomy 21?

There is an interesting side story to the discovery of trisomy 21 as the cause of DS. In 2009, the fiftieth anniversary of the paper by Lejeune, Gauthier, and Turpin, Lejeune's colleague and coauthor, Marie Gauthier, wrote a paper claiming that she was the one who actually made the discovery.[18] According to Gauthier's quite personal and detailed account, it was she, not Lejeune, who did the cytogenetics, she who set up a lab in Paris, and she who found the extra chromosome in the cells of children with DS. Lejeune, according to her account, took her slides, hid them from her, claimed credit for the discovery, and never acknowledged that the original work was hers. Gauthier wrote,

I entrusted the slides to J. L., who had the photos taken but did not show them to me; they were, he said, with the Chief and therefore under lock and key. I was too young to know the rules of the game. I suspected political manoeuvring, and I was not wrong. Reporting for the CNRS at the Ionising Radiation Congress in Canada, and without planning anything with Turpin or indeed with me, he mentioned the discovery at a McGill seminar in October 1958 as though he were its author. Contrary to standard practice, J. L. signed first and my name only appears second. As usual, Prof. Turpin, the leader responsible for the initial hypothesis, signed last. I was hurt and suspected a degree of manipulation, having a feeling of being the "forgotten discoverer."

J. L. then whipped up a great storm in the media, being interviewed by all the papers. J. L. was then showered with all kinds of rewards, being promoted from CNRS trainee to master of research and winning a gold medal. Progressively, through his participation in numerous congresses, he was hailed as the only discoverer and ended up convincing himself of that, to such an extent that Prof. Turpin's descendants kicked up a fuss through their lawyers. In addition, they lodged in the Pasteur Institute's archives their father's articles certifying his seniority in the chromosome-based hypothesis concerning mongolism, which was finally verified.

This sordid story of one scientist claiming recognition he does not deserve while another scientist fails to receive the recognition that she does deserve is of course not unique. Gauthier herself notes this when she compares herself to Johann Friedrich Miescher, who discovered DNA,[19] or Rosalind Franklin, who figured out its molecular structure.[20] The story of Lejeune's discovery, his fame, and the uses to which he put that fame are an important chapter in the modern history of childbirth. Lejeune is a morally complex figure. He used the fame that he achieved by claiming credit for a discovery he did not make in order to advocate for an approach to prenatal care that reflected his deeply held Christian beliefs.

The Legacy of Liley and Lejeune

Liley's pioneering work in amniocentesis would be coupled with Lejeune's work in cytogenetics to develop new ways to diagnose fetal anomalies. Using amniocentesis, clinicians could obtain samples of amniotic fluid that contained cells from the fetus. These cells could be grown in tissue culture, the chromosomes isolated, and prenatal diagnoses of chromosomal anomalies made.

Taken together, these discoveries allowed a change in the way we think about the appropriate age at which women should bear children. The older a woman is when she conceives a baby, the higher the likelihood of a chromosomal anomaly. Among pregnant women who are 30 years of age, DS affects only 1 in 1000 fetuses. By age 35, it is three times more common. For pregnant women who are 40, DS is present in one of every 100 pregnancies.[21] Prior to the development of amniocentesis, many women hesitated to have babies once they turned 30 or 35 in order to avoid the increasing risks of such problems. The techniques of prenatal diagnosis, coupled with the legalization of abortion, allowed women to postpone childbearing without facing the relatively high risk of having a baby with DS or other chromosomal anomalies. So amniocentesis and prenatal diagnosis play a key role in the story we tell in later chapters about trends in the age distribution of childbearing.

But the discoveries and innovations of Liley and Lejeune had further implications. They changed forever the way we think about prenatal care. Following their lead, obstetricians developed many ways of assessing the health and well-being of the fetus. These include prenatal ultrasound, chorionic villus biopsy, intrauterine fetal monitoring, fetal magnetic resonance imaging, and blood tests on pregnant women that can be used to screen for anomalies in the fetus. Surgeons experimented with in utero maternal-fetal surgery for congenital anomalies. Each of these innovations allowed a more fine-grained and accurate assessment of the health of the fetus. They catalyzed the transformation of prenatal care from an endeavor designed primarily to monitor and promote the health of the pregnant woman to one designed not only to take care of the mother but also to monitor and promote the health of the fetus.

Intrauterine transfusions would lead to the development of ultrasound as a way of guiding the intrauterine transfusion devices. Ultrasound allowed the diagnosis of anatomical abnormalities and eventually to screening tests for chromosomal anomalies. In utero diagnosis of anatomical abnormalities would lead to in utero surgery in an attempt to correct many of these abnormalities. It also allowed more accurate assessment of gestational age. This, in turn, became a guide for obstetricians as they tried to decide the relative risks and benefits of medically induced preterm birth, given how much easier it is to carry out medical interventions on an infant outside the womb compared to inside.

Prenatal care as we know it today is something very different from what it was before the work of Bevis, Liley, Lejeune, Nadler, and others. Before we turn to an analysis of the impact that these changes in prenatal care have had on the rate of preterm birth, we need to examine two other phenomena that are an important part of the story of the ways that childbearing has changed in the last half century. One is the development of the birth control pill. This allowed women to control their fertility, to delay childbirth, and to pursue advanced education and more ambitious career paths before they bore children. The other, related issue is the effect that delayed childbearing has had on the rate of preterm birth.

10 The Pill (and Delayed Childbearing)

The oral contraceptive pill may not seem to be part of the story about prenatal care and preterm birth. But it is an essential part. The development of a safe and effective oral contraceptive pill allowed women to have, for the first time in human history, reliable control over their fertility without the need of any cooperation from their sexual partners. They could choose when they would have babies.

The first oral contraceptive pill was a combination of two hormones, norethynodrel and mestranol, marketed under the brand name Enovid. It was approved by the U.S. Food and Drug Administration in 1957 for the treatment of gynecologic disorders, primarily dysmenorrhea and irregular menses. Between 1957 and 1960, its safety and efficacy as a contraceptive had been tested in 830 Puerto Rican and Haitian women.[1] The pill proved to be almost 100% effective in preventing pregnancy. The few failures were attributed to noncompliance rather than imperfect efficacy. In May of 1960, the FDA approved its use as an oral contraceptive.

The pill quickly found a large market. Fourteen percent of new patients at Planned Parenthood clinics in 1961 chose to use oral contraceptives for birth control. By 1964 that number had jumped to 62%.[2] The pill's popularity was based not only on its efficacy but also on its convenience. It did not need to be used at the time of sexual activity. It did not require any cooperation or acquiescence by the man. It was not cumbersome. Its use could be secret.

With the power and control given to them by the pill, many women opted to delay childbearing. Women today have babies at older ages than they did in the past. The percentage of births to women under 25 has drifted steadily downward. More women are having babies in their late thirties or early forties.[3]

That change was not entirely a direct result of the pill; many other social changes were taking place at the same time. But the availability of the pill is a part of the complex story. It had a powerful effect on women's reproductive decisions, and thereby on their inextricably related career and life decisions.

Though it is impossible to summarize the effect that the birth control pill had on society, it is probably not an exaggeration to say that the pill changed forever the ways that people think about sex, marriage, and women's biological destiny. It changed the ways that women thought about their own bodies, their relationships with men, their careers, and their life goals.

These claims may seem grandiose. After all, the oral contraceptive was introduced at a time of sweeping social change. The pill was both a result of these changes and a catalyst for many of them. We can track the temporal associations between the usage of oral contraception and, say, college graduation rates, average age at childbearing, fertility, and other statistics. Still, it is hard to know whether, or to what degree, the pill caused or accelerated those changes in women's lives or, by contrast, to what extent those changes were simply concurrent with the introduction of oral contraception and reflected broader underlying social changes.

There is some evidence that the pill itself, and not other social changes, catalyzed changes in women's career choices. The evidence comes from studies of changes in the percentages of women who finished college and went on to graduate or professional schools in the years after the pill first became available. And it is possible to analyze this relationship in the United States because state laws differed as to whether they allowed college students to obtain the pill.

Before the late 1960s, it was technically illegal throughout the United States for a physician to prescribe contraceptives to an unmarried woman. (This did not, of course, stop some women from getting oral contraceptives. Some got around the law by claiming that they were engaged to be married. Others claimed that the purpose of the pills was to regulate irregular menstrual periods.[4])

The legislative changes that led to unhindered and legal access to contraceptives for unmarried women occurred in different states at different times during the 1960s and 1970s. In 1965, in most states, minors could not obtain contraceptives without parental permission. In 1969, the age of majority for women was 21 in most states. But in six states (Alaska, Kentucky, Nevada, Oklahoma, Utah, and Idaho) the age of majority was 18. Three states (California, Georgia, and Mississippi) allowed "mature minors" to obtain contraception without parental permission. By 1974, most states had changed their policies. With the change, university health services began providing oral contraceptive pills. In 1966, according to the American College Health Association, just 3.6% of colleges provided the pill to unmarried students.[5] By 1973, 19% of colleges did so; because these were mostly larger colleges, 42% of undergraduates in the United States could easily obtain the pill.

Goldin and Katz use the state-to-state variations in access to the pill to examine the effect of the pill on women's completion of college and graduate school.[6] They begin their analysis by noting that "the availability of family planning services to women *when they are in college* is a critical input to career change because it occurs when career, marriage, and family decisions are being made. The point is central to our analysis since access to the pill was not a major issue for most women after they were in professional and graduate school."

They then take advantage of the "natural experiment" that occurred in the United States in the late 1960s and early 1970s when different states applied different policies governing access to the pill for unmarried college students. The researchers could thus analyze the impact of state laws regarding birth control access for minors on a variety of outcomes, including the likelihood of getting married before age 23 and the percentage of women enrolled in professional schools. They analyze this by state for college-educated women born in the United States from 1935 to 1957, that is, for women who would have started college between 1953 and 1975. They control for access to abortion (abortion bans were repealed in five states in 1970 and everywhere in 1973 with *Roe v. Wade*).

The data and conclusions of Goldin and Katz are striking. They first report general trends. "Women were 10 percent of first-year law students in 1970 but 36% in 1980. Among the cohort of female college graduates born in 1950, almost 50 percent married before age 23, but fewer than 30 percent did for those born in 1957."[7] They then show that these changes were associated with access to the pill. Wherever the pill became available, women were more likely to finish college, less likely to be married before the age of 23, and more likely to go on to graduate or professional schools.

The pill was not, of course, the only factor involved in these changes. But, the authors note, "a virtually foolproof, easy-to-use, and female-controlled contraceptive having low health risks, little pain, and few annoyances does appear to have been important in promoting real change in the economic status of women."

Birdsall and Chester came to similar conclusions. In a review and analysis of the effect of the pill that they published in 1987, they noted that, while it is impossible to establish direct causation, much data supports the view that "progression toward near-perfect control over childbearing has probably contributed to marked changes in the education and employment patterns of U.S. women over the past two decades."[8]

To be clear: the pill may not have directly caused the changes in women's lives. It may have merely been associated with them. For example, states that gave minors access to contraceptives might have other policies or prevalent attitudes that affected young women's decisions. But for the main concerns of this book, it doesn't really matter whether the pill was a cause of change, one of many causes of change, or merely a symbol of change. It was one of the new technologies that allowed a dramatic shift in the ways that women thought about childbearing within their overall life course.

The pill generated much moral controversy. But contraception has always been controversial. About one hundred years ago, on October 16, 1916, Margaret Sanger opened the first birth control clinic in the United States. Sanger's Brooklyn clinic stayed open for ten days before police raided the clinic and arrested Sanger and her sister, Ethel Byrne, for violating the New York state law by which it was a misdemeanor to give away or sell contraceptive information. Sanger's defense challenged the constitutionality of that state law. The trial judge rejected her arguments, but an appeals court ruled that contraceptives could be sold to prevent disease. Following that decision, condom manufacturers marked their products as useful "for the prevention of disease only." Their business thrived. In 1938, *Fortune* magazine pronounced birth control one of the most prosperous businesses of the decade; it had racked up more than $250 million in annual sales.[9]

The legal availability of contraception allowed women some control over their fertility. And they used it. Between 1880 and 1940, long before the pill, women's average fertility rate (that is, the total number of babies they had during their lifetime) in the United States dropped by over 50%. For white women, it dropped from 4.4 children per woman to 2.1. For black women, it dropped from 7.5 children to 3.0.[10] But the most common forms of birth control—condoms, diaphragms, vaginal douches, and intrauterine devices of one sort or another—were unwieldy and not completely reliable.

Sanger was an early advocate for research on a birth control pill. She dreamed of a form of birth control that would give women full control over their fertility without the cooperation of their male partners.[11] There was no government support for such a project. In fact, in many states, such research was banned. Sanger found an ally and a funder in the philanthropist Katharine Dexter McCormick, heir to the fortune of Cyrus McCormick, founder of the International Harvester Company. Over her lifetime, McCormick gave more than $2 million to the research that led to the development of the contraceptive pill. Most of that money went to support the research of Gregory Pincus and the Worcester Foundation for Experimental Biology.

Many books have recounted the complex history of the development of oral contraceptives.[12-16] A PBS documentary summed up the story like this: "Among the key players in the development of the drug were two elderly female activists who demanded a contraceptive women could eat like aspirin and then paid for the scientific research; a devout Catholic gynecologist who believed a robust sex life made for a good marriage and argued tirelessly that the Pill was a natural form of birth control; and a brilliant biologist who bullied a pharmaceutical company into risking a possibly crippling boycott to develop this revolutionary contraceptive."[17] At every stage along the way there were legal, ethical, and religious controversies. Some of the controversies faded. Others continue to this day and remain salient issues in national politics.

Doctors argued about whether contraception itself was good or bad for women's health, and, if so, whether the risks outweighed the benefits of preventing pregnancy.[18] Feminists argued about whether the pill liberated women from biological destiny or whether, instead, it was just another example of patriarchal medical control over women's bodies.[19] A search of the National Library of Medicine database using the key words "risk" and "oral contraceptive" yields over 10,000 articles.[20] The PBS film history noted:

After a decade on the market, the wonder drug that had been lauded by women as "liberating" and "revolutionary" came under attack by feminists. Senate hearings in 1970 brought the health risks of the Pill to the attention of the nation. Many women were furious. Feminists now saw the Pill as yet another example of patriarchal control over women's lives. Women's disillusionment with the Pill fed into the new feminist critique of American society. Women started asking questions such as: Why should birth control be a female responsibility? Why do men control the medical profession and the pharmaceutical industry? Do women's health interests suffer as a result? For a growing number of women, the Pill was proof positive that the personal was political.[21]

Two aspects of the widespread availability and use of oral contraceptives are relevant to the changes that took place in prenatal care and preterm birth. First, the introduction of the pill was associated with delayed childbearing and, in particular, with delayed childbearing for the purpose of starting careers. Second, the choice to delay childbearing would have been associated with a higher risk of fetal anomalies unless women also had access to prenatal diagnosis and legal abortion.

If delayed childbearing had led to much higher incidence of Down syndrome and other chromosomal anomalies, the pill's effectiveness probably would not have resulted in so many women choosing that option. Women would have been more reluctant to delay childbearing for long if not for the availability of amniocentesis and prenatal diagnosis. And these new techniques wouldn't have been very useful if not for another huge change in law and public policy, the legalization of abortion. We will talk more about abortion in later chapters, but first we review the statistics on delayed childbearing along with other changes in the demographics of childbirth.

11   The Changing Demography of Childbearing

In this chapter, we will present a possibly mind-numbing collection of statistics to show how the demographics of childbearing in the United States have changed over the last forty years. We do so for three reasons. First, we want to make the case that delayed childbearing is just one of a number of changes that might affect the rate of preterm birth. Second, we want to set the stage for our analysis in the next chapter of the net effect of all these changes on the rate of preterm birth. In that analysis, we analyze the degree to which the changes in the demographics of childbearing contributed to our high rate of preterm birth. The third reason is that the issues surrounding delayed childbearing bear directly on the case we have been presenting and following, our 34-year-old with infertility problems who's experiencing a somewhat problematic pregnancy. Below, we will analyze how much of the rise in preterm birth is related to similar cases.

There are three different ways to measure the fertility of a population. One is to look at the total number of births in a population each year. Another is to look at the average number of babies that each woman has over the course of her lifetime. A third is to look at the number of babies born per year to all women of childbearing age.

In 2007, there were more births in the United States—about 4.3 million—than ever before. It is about the same number of babies as were born at the height of the baby boom in 1957. After 1957, the total number of babies born fell steadily—to 4 million in 1964, then to 3.1 million in 1973. Then the number began to rise again, slowly and steadily, to its recent high level. After 2007, it slowly dropped again. In 2012, there were about 3.9 million births.

While the total number of babies born is at a near record high, the average number of births to each woman in the United States is near an all-time low. However, it is not an unprecedented low. Like the total number of births, it is a number we have seen before. In 1900, women averaged about 3.5 children over their lifetime. During the depression of the 1930s, the annual rate fell so dramatically that, had a woman experienced that rate throughout her childbearing years, she would have had, on average, only about 2 babies over her lifetime. The rate rose again after World War II and peaked in 1960, at an average of 3.65 babies per woman. Then it began to fall steadily once again. In 2007, the number was similar to that seen during the Great Depression, 2.1.[1] It has remained there since. That number is high compared to other industrialized countries. In most European countries, women have on average fewer than 2 babies during their lifetime—a rate that, without immigration, leads to declining population.[2]

The *fertility rate* is the number of births per year for every 1,000 women between the ages of 15 and 44. One hundred years ago, the fertility rate in the United States was 125 per 1,000. That is, about one in every 8 women of childbearing age had a baby each year. By 1950, the rate had fallen to 106, or about one in 10 women. This decline in fertility began before the so-called sexual revolution and before the availability of the birth control pill.[3] Fertility fell further, to about 70 per 1,000 by 1980, and has remained about the same since then. (In 2007, it was down to 69.5.) In other words, today, about 1 of every 14 women of child-bearing age in the United States has a baby every year.

Fertility rates are based upon births, not pregnancies. We can also measure total numbers of pregnancies and classify those that end by induced abortion or by miscarriage or stillbirth. On average, about 60% to 65% of pregnancies result in a live birth. The rates of induced abortion rose after 1973. They peaked in 1981 at 29% of all pregnancies. Since then, that percentage has steadily fallen. In 1990, 24% of pregnancies ended with an induced abortion. In 2011, that rate had fallen to 17%.[4] Rates of known miscarriage have risen slightly, from 15% to 17%.[5]

To summarize, there are more women in the United States now than ever. Those women are having fewer babies, on average, than did women in the past. Because there are more people, there are more births, even though each woman is having fewer babies.

These trends are worth discussing for two reasons. First, they suggest just how malleable the birth rate is and has been throughout the twentieth century. People have always made decisions about whether and when to have babies. Control over fertility did not start with the birth control pill or the legalization of abortion. The low fertility rate in the 1930s demonstrates that mechanisms for limiting childbearing were as available in the 1930s as in the 1960s, on a population level. The big change in the 1960s, associated with the birth control pill, was that it became possible for each woman to reliably control her own fertility and to turn it off or on when she wanted. The dip in fertility during the Great Depression suggests, too, the important role played by economic factors in decisions about childbearing. People have children when they can afford them, and don't have them when they cannot. At least that used to be the case.

Second, the more recent trends suggest that, today, the decision-making dynamic for decisions about whether and when to have babies is different than it had been in the past. Such decisions used to be linked to economic cycles. When the economy was good, people had more babies. That no longer seems to be the case. In the 1980s and 1990s, people were having fewer babies in spite of economic prosperity. The recession that began in 2007 has led to a slight decrease in the total number of births. But that drop was only a small one. To use the language of economists, the demand for babies has become quite inelastic. People seem to know how many babies they want to have over the course of their lives, and it appears that they set out to have precisely that number of babies. They are more or less able to have those babies at the time in their lives when they want. Thus, we have seen the triumph of a "planned parenthood" approach, in the generic rather than the proprietary sense of that term. This is true even though, in individual cases, planning may not be perfect. There are still many unplanned pregnancies, and there are many women who want to get pregnant and cannot. But, overall, people can and do exercise much more control than they did in the past.

Buried in these overall fertility trends are some interesting shifts in the subgroups of women who are having babies. Two big shifts are especially important to the question of preterm birth. One is a shift in the ethnicity and immigrant status of women who are having babies. A higher proportion of babies are born to Hispanic and foreign-born mothers than ever before. In 1990, 15% of all births in the United States were to women who had been born outside the United States. In 2004, the percentage of births to foreign-born mothers peaked at 24% of all births in the United States.[6] Since then it has fallen slightly.[7]

The other big demographic shift is in the age of women who are having babies. Women in their teens and twenties are having fewer babies. Women in their thirties and forties are having more. The average age at childbearing has been rising for the last forty years. The mean age of women *at the time of their first birth* increased by nearly four years between 1968 and 2002, from 21.4 to 25.1 years of age. Over those same years the *average age at childbearing* rose from 24.9 to 27.3.[8]

This trend toward higher maternal age at the time of childbirth is partly accounted for by higher rates of pregnancy in older women. It is also a result of lower rates of pregnancy in teens. The rate of teen pregnancy has been falling steadily over the last forty years. In 1970, nearly 40% of women had their first baby before age 20. In 2012, the number of babies born to teenagers in the United States was lower than it has been since World War II.[9]

Since 1980, the percentage of first pregnancies to women over the age of 35 in the United States has more than quadrupled, from less than 1% to more than 4%. Black, Hispanic, and Native American women tend to have their first babies at younger ages than non-Hispanic White women in the United States.

Another way to characterize these trends is to examine the fertility rates for women at different ages. Between 1990 and 2004, the fertility rate dropped dramatically for teenagers and for women aged 20 to 24. It dropped slightly for women 25 to 29. It rose for women who were 30 or older, with the biggest rise for women over 35.[10]

Figure 11.1 illustrates some of the changes in the demography of childbearing in the United States between 1990 and 2010.

The rate of pregnancy in unmarried women has risen steadily. This trend has been apparent since at least 1940, when only about 5% of births in U.S. were to unmarried women. In 2012, 41% of U.S. births were to unmarried women.[11]

Poor women have the highest fertility rates, with a steady drop as economic status rises.[12] The fertility rate for women in families with an annual income below $10,000 is 87 per 1,000. It is lower—79 per 1,000—for women with family incomes of

Number of births, by mothers' characteristics, 1990 and 2010

	1990			2010		
	All	U.S. born	Foreign born	All	U.S. born	Foreign born
All births	4,158,212	3,504,640	645,589	3,999,386	3,055,817	930,135
White	2,626,500	2,512,837	110,581	2,162,406	2,024,558	132,745
Black	661,701	614,123	44,927	589,808	507,138	78,326
Hispanic	595,073	230,587	363,684	945,180	418,237	525,319
Asian	134,837	18,965	115,696	234,472	46,291	186,945
Mexican	385,640	146,978	238,269	598,317	251,650	346,113
NonMexican	3,772,572	3,357,662	407,320	3,401,069	2,804,167	584,022
Younger than 20	533,483	472,705	59,163	372,175	324,452	46,077
20–34	3,256,901	2,737,429	513,690	3,047,571	2,345,790	692,117
35 and older	367,828	294,506	72,736	579,640	385,575	191,941
Married	2,992,828	2,518,497	471,290	2,365,915	1,763,221	596,933
Unmarried	1,165,384	986,143	174,299	1,633,471	1,292,596	333,202

Figure 11.1

Some changes in the demographics of childbearing in the United States, 1990–2010. Data from the Centers for Disease Control and Prevention National Vital Statistics System. http://www.cdc.gov/nchs/nvss/cohort_fertility_tables.htm

$25,000 to $29,000. For women in families with incomes over $75,000, the fertility rate is 60 per 1,000.

Among the major racial and ethnic groups, in 2007, fertility rates were highest for Hispanic women (102 per 1,000) and lowest for non-Hispanic white women (60 per 1,000).[13]

Each of these shifts over time could have an effect on the rate of preterm birth. Older women, as we discuss in the next chapter, are more likely to have preterm births. Blacks have higher rates of preterm births than Whites. Hispanic women, particularly immigrants, have lower rates of preterm birth than Blacks. Teens are at higher risk for preterm birth than are women in their twenties.

In order to sort out the effects of all these demographic changes, we designed a study to estimate what the rate of preterm birth would have been in 2005 if the demography of childbearing had not changed from what it was in 1985. We present the methodology and the results in chapter 15. First, however, we review the data on the effects of childbearing at older ages on preterm birth and fertility rates.

12 Maternal Age, Multiple Pregnancies, and Preterm Birth

The rise in average age at childbearing is associated with many good outcomes. Teen pregnancy is associated with higher risks of pregnancy complications, so outcomes are better when there are fewer teens having babies. Older women are more likely to have higher incomes, to have planned their pregnancies, and to have social support.

But delayed childbearing also increases some risks. Older age at childbearing is associated with higher rates of preterm birth, stillbirth, and multiple gestations. Older women are also more likely to have problems with fertility, and treatment for fertility is in turn associated with pregnancy complications. We will discuss IVF below, but first we review the data on problems associated with childbearing at older ages.

The data on maternal age and the risk of preterm birth comes from large demographic studies of birth outcomes conducted in many different countries over many recent time periods. Cnattingius and colleagues studied all singleton first births in Sweden between 1983 and 1987. They compared outcomes for women 20 to 24 years of age with those of women 30 to 34, 35 to 39, and 40 or older. They found that older women had significantly higher rates of preterm birth, low birthweight babies, and intrauterine fetal deaths.[1] Astolfi and colleagues conducted a similar study in Italy and found similar results: the risk of preterm birth was 30% higher for women in their early thirties, compared to those in their twenties. For women in their late thirties, the risk was almost twice as high as for women in their twenties.[2] Aldous and Edmonson found similar results in the state of Washington.[3] Tough and colleagues examined birth records in the Canadian province of Alberta between the years 1990 and 1996. During those years, the percentage of babies born to women over 35 years of age rose 51%, from 8.4% to 12.6% of births in the province. They showed that, as the average age at childbearing increased, the rate of low birthweight and preterm birth also rose. Some of this was accounted for by a rise in multiples. The rate of twin pregnancies was 15% higher in women over 35 than in younger women. There were 14% more triplet pregnancies. Tough and colleagues calculated that changes in maternal age at childbirth accounted for 78% of the change in low birthweight rate in Alberta and 36% of the change in preterm delivery rate in the population.[4]

Higher maternal age is also associated with an increased risk of stillbirth. Huang and colleagues summarized 37 studies of different populations and showed that older maternal age was significantly associated with greater risk of stillbirth. The degree of risk is difficult to pinpoint. The increased risk of stillbirth for older mothers compared to younger mothers ranged from 20% to 250% across different study populations.[5]

The reasons behind the high rates of preterm birth and still-birth among older women are only partially understood. It may be related to overall health. The incidence of most chronic medical problems increases with age and so it is not surprising that older mothers tend to have more medical problems, including hypertension, diabetes, and obesity, compared to younger mothers.[6] They are more likely to have multiple pregnancies (i.e., twins, triplets, etc.), and multiple pregnancies at any age are associated with preterm birth.[7] There is an ongoing debate about whether maternal age is simply a marker for other health conditions that are associated with preterm birth or whether age itself is an independent risk factor. One review of this debate concluded, "There is insufficient evidence to determine if older maternal age is an independent and direct risk factor for preterm birth and SGA [small for gestational age] birth, or a risk marker that exerts its influence on gestational age or birth weight or both through its association with age-dependent confounders. Future research is needed to quantify the independent impact of delayed childbearing on neonatal outcomes, as well as to identify the pathways involved."[8]

It is likely that the rise in preterm birth rates among women who have delayed childbearing into their thirties and forties results from a combination of factors, including the ones noted here as well as others that have not yet been discovered. For some of these factors, such as diabetes, prevention or treatment might be effective. For others, such as the rise in multiples or the poorly understood "independent effect" of age, better health behaviors or better medical care are unlikely to help. In either case, the association of higher maternal age and higher rates of preterm birth is likely to persist.

13 Maternal Age and Infertility

Higher maternal age is associated with higher rates of infertility.[1] That fact is well known. It is less well known exactly when or how fast the risk of infertility problems rises. The data are complex because, as one review noted, "One of the limitations of previous studies of 'How late can you wait?' is that any observed decline in the probability of conception with age could be due to a decline in fecundability with age or due to a decline in coital frequency with age or due to both factors."[2] In addition, the likelihood of having a baby depends on both successful conception and successful gestation. These two features of female reproductive capacity do not decline at the same rate.

Inability to conceive is categorized as "primary infertility," and it increases with each decade. Among women aged 15 to 24 in the United States, 4.4% reported that they were unable to conceive after a year of trying. In the 25 to 34 age group, 6.6% of women were infertile by the same definition. For women 35 to 44, the rate was 8.0%.[3]

The infertility associated with age is amenable to intervention. The treatments, however, carry risks. Broadly speaking, there are two types of treatments for primary infertility: drugs that stimulate ovulation and in vitro fertilization (IVF).

National data on the use of drugs to stimulate ovulation are not available from the United States. Such data have been reported from other places. In British Columbia, a relatively high use locale, ovarian stimulants are used by 4.5 women per 1,000 between the ages of 30 and 44.[4] The rates are similar in the Netherlands.[5] Among women over 30, there has been a steady increase in the use of clomiphene, one of the most widely used ovarian stimulants.

There are about 61 million women of childbearing age in the United States, and about 25 million are between 30 and 44. If the U.S. rate of clomiphene use is similar to that in the Netherlands and in British Columbia, approximately 500,000 to 750,000 women per year use that (or similar) medication.

We have excellent data on IVF because all cases are reported to the Centers for Disease Control. In 2010, there were a total of 147,260 attempts at in vitro fertilization. A total of 61,564 infants born in the United States that year were conceived using IVF.[6] That is between 1% and 2% of all births.

Both IVF and ovulation-inducing drugs are associated with increased rates of preterm birth. This occurs in two ways. Both IVF and ovarian stimulation are associated with higher rates of twins and triplets, which are born preterm at a much higher rate. In addition, even singleton pregnancies that follow IVF are more likely to result in preterm birth than are pregnancies that did not require IVF.

Taken together, the combination of delayed childbearing and more treatment for infertility has led to a dramatic and unprecedented rise in multiple pregnancies over the last three decades. In 1981, twin pregnancies accounted for 19.3 of every 1,000, and only 0.4 per 1,000 pregnancies were triplets or higher-order multiples. By 2007, 32.2 out of 1,000 pregnancies were twin pregnancies, and 1.5 in 1,000 were triplets or more. Thus, over those 26 years the rate of twin pregnancies rose 67% and the rate of triplets almost quadrupled.

About 40% of the rise in multiple pregnancies has been attributed to either IVF or ovulation-inducing drugs. The percentage attributable to IVF is more precisely known, because all IVF centers report results to the CDC. Of 52,792 infants who were conceived using IVF in 2006, nearly 26,000 were multiples. Thus, IVF accounted for 17% of all twins and 38% of higher-order multiples that year. The contribution of ovulation-inducing drugs is harder to calculate. Schieve and Devine used a complex analytic algorithm to estimate this impact.[7] They concluded that, in 2005, about 23% of multiple births in the United States were attributable to ovulation-inducing drugs. More recently, Kulkarni and colleagues estimated that "the proportion of twin births resulting from medically assisted conceptions rose from 27% in 1998 to 36% in 2011. The estimated proportion of twin births that were attributable to non-IVF fertility treatments increased from 16% in 1998 to 19% in 2011 (a statistically significant change), and the estimated proportion of triplet and higher-order births attributable to non-IVF fertility treatments increased from 36% in 1998 to 45% in 2011."[8] Taken together, then, IVF and ovulation-inducing drugs account for nearly half of the increase in multiple gestations in the United States. What accounts for the rest of the rise in multiples? Even in the absence of fertility treatments, older age is associated with increased rates of multiples. The CDC estimates that about one-third of the increase in twins in the three decades since 1980 is due to increased maternal age.[9] Many twins and almost all higher-order multiples are born preterm, so this rise in multiples, due to older maternal age (both directly and indirectly through fertility treatments), also contributes to the rise in preterm birth rates.

We can estimate the relative contribution of infertility treatments to preterm birth rates. The rate of preterm birth rose from about 8% in 1980 to about 12% today. (That number includes both singletons and multiple pregnancies.) There are about 4 million births per year in the United States, so there were about 320,000 preterm births in 1980 and about 480,000 by 2007. At the beginning of that time period, infertility treatment was uncommon, so we can assume that very few of the preterm births were attributable to such treatment in 1980. By the end of the time period, IVF accounted for 21,000 preemies.[10] Ovulation-stimulating drugs probably accounted for slightly more. So, taken together, infertility treatments may have accounted for 10% of preterm deliveries, or about 25% of the increase in preterm births.

To summarize, the net effect of delayed childbearing on preterm birth rates is a combination of the higher rate of preterm delivery associated with increasing maternal age, the higher rate of infertility leading to infertility treatment, and the risks of preterm birth associated with such treatments. To those underlying risks, one must add yet another risk factor. Because older women are at higher risk than younger women for preterm birth, they are monitored more closely during prenatal care. Closer monitoring increases the probability of finding problems that will lead to a medically induced preterm delivery.

Delayed childbearing is, of course, only one of many demographic changes that could have affected the preterm birth rate over the last thirty years. The next chapter discusses some of the other changes.

14 Changing Demography and Preterm Birth Rates

Many discussions of the rising rate of preterm birth start with the assumption that rising maternal age, with accompanying infertility, infertility treatment, and multiple births, is one of the primary underlying causes. A study of preterm birth trends in Canada from 1981 through 1994 came to this conclusion. Researchers showed that "substantial increases in the rates of preterm births have occurred among births resulting from multiple gestation, concurrently with increases in the frequency of multiple births."[1] They suggested that the rise in multiples was associated with delayed childbearing and a resultant rise in infertility and infertility treatment.

Another study examining this phenomenon in Canada, England and Wales, France, and the United States found similar results. The authors write:

In 1981 to 1997, the rate of twins increased by 28% to 45% in each country. The increases in triplet rates were even more dramatic: 358% in the United States, 273% in England and Wales, 197% in Canada, and 111% in France. In 1995 to 1997, the preterm birth rate in Canada was 11% higher than that for 1981 to 1983, and the U.S. rate was 15% higher. Singleton preterm delivery rates were under 10% in 1995 to 1997; however, the rates for twins were nearly 50%, and those for triplets were over 90%. The increases in rates of both twins and triplets in each country reflect, to some extent, the rising maternal age at childbirth observed in most developed countries, given that multiple-birth rates are higher for older women. It has been estimated that between a quarter and a third of the increase in twin and triplet deliveries can be attributed to the increase in maternal age.[2]

These studies look at one aspect of the changing demography of childbirth. But they ignore other ways that the changing demographics of childbearing might influence the preterm birth rate. At the same time as the rise in the number of births to women in their thirties and forties, there has been an decrease in births to teens, a rise in births to immigrant mothers, a decrease in births to mothers who received no prenatal care, a rise in births to unmarried women, and many other changes in our demographic patterns of childbearing.

We wanted to know how much of the increase in the preterm birth rate is due to changes in the demographic characteristics of childbearing women. Unfortunately, an unambiguous answer would require that we live a reality that cannot exist; that we see how many preterm births there would be in today's world of obstetric practice if the characteristics of childbearing women had not changed in recent decades. We designed a study that statistically mimics that unobservable reality. We collaborated with the biostatistician Tyler VanderWeele and designed a statistical model that would allow us to test the following counterfactual question: "What changes would we have seen in the rates of preterm birth in the United States if the demography of childbearing had not changed since 1989?" In other words, how much of the observed rise in preterm birth can be explained either by changes in maternal factors related to preterm birth, such as age, race, education, marital status, and nativity, or by the increase in the number of multiple pregnancies.[3]

To do this, we used the files that include all of birth certificates in the country each year. These files are prepared by the National Center for Health Statistics (NCHS) for research purposes and include all of the information on birth certificates except those data elements that could be used to identify individuals. Because there have been changes in how data were collected on birth certificates over the years, we focused on the 15-year period from 1989 to 2004, a period with fairly comparable birth certificate data and also a period that saw an increase in preterm birth rates and sizable changes in the demography of mothers and in the rates of multiples. Preterm birth was categorized according to the gestational-age variable in the NCHS data, derived from the last menstrual period (LMP). Gestational age less than 37 weeks was considered preterm. We further used the delivery character-istics information to categorize each preterm birth as "spontane-ous" or as "medically induced." The data on the birth certificate are not ideal for this determination, but the same approach has been used in the research literature. Medically induced preterm was defined as a delivery by C-section or with induction prior to 37 weeks. The limitation is that it is possible that some of the deliveries by C-section or induction actually followed a spontaneous but ineffective labor. The other characteristics of the mother and pregnancy that we considered were age, race/ ethnicity, education, marital status, birth history, maternal place of birth, and geographic division of the country). Singleton or multiple births were sorted into three categories: single, twin, and triplet or higher.

We compared preterm birth rates, maternal characteristics, and multiple pregnancies between 1989 and 2004. From 1989 to 2004, preterm births increased from 11.2% of all births to 12.8% of all births, a 14% increase. Some of the comparisons were surprising. From 1989 to 2004, the rate of spontaneous preterm births actually declined by 20%, from 7.8% of all births to 6.2%, The increase in preterm birth was entirely accounted for by medically induced preterm births. The rate of medically induced preterm births nearly doubled over those years, from 3.4% to 6.6% of all births. Furthermore, the rise in medically induced preterm births occurred in roughly the same proportion in all demographic categories. It occurred among women who were younger or older, women with singletons or multiples, women who were born in the United States and those who had immigrated.

There were changes in most of the maternal demographic factors. The age distribution of mothers had shifted to older ages. For example, the percentage of births to teen mothers declined from 12.6% to 10.2%. At the other end of the age distribution, the percentage of births to mothers 35 and older increased from 8.6% to 14.4% of all births. The percentage of births to Hispanic mothers increased from 13% to 23% while the percentage to non-Hispanic white mothers declined from 66% to 57%. The percentage of mothers with 16 years or more of schooling increased from 18% to 27% while the percentage with just 12 years fell by ten percent. The percentage of mothers who were unmarried increased from 27% to 35% and the percentage of mothers born in the United States declined from 85% to 76%. Altogether, these are dramatic changes for a 15-year period. In addition, the percentage of births that were twins increased by about 40% and the percentage that were higher-order multiples increased by about 250%.

Next we determined the risk of preterm birth for every combination of predictive factors in 2004, and we applied those risks to the actual women in 1989 to estimate what the preterm birth rate would be for 2004 if the demographic characteristics of the mothers looked the same as in 1989. Surprisingly, the percentage who were predicted to deliver preterm was exactly the same as the actual 2004 rate: 12.8%.

Similar analyses examined spontaneous and medically induced preterm birth considered separately, and added multiple births as a covariate in the statistical models in order to examine whether trends in preterm birth rates (overall, spontaneous, or medically induced) were further explained by changes in multiple births from 1989 to 2004.

When all factors were taken into account, the actual 2004 rates of both spontaneous and medically induced preterm birth were exactly the same as the "counterfactual" rates. About 16% of the increase in the rate of medically induced preterm birth is explained by increased multiple births.

The results suggest that the rise in preterm birth in the United States between 1989 and 2004 was not a result of the changing demography of childbearing. It was not simply the result of delayed childbearing, more infertility, and more multiple pregnancies leading to more medically induced preterm births, although multiples play a small role. Instead, these data show that the rise in preterm births is a result of changes in obstetric practice. Simply put, there are more medically induced preterm births—that is, cesarean deliveries and medical inductions of labor—in all demographic groups. The proportion of such births in both high-risk and low-risk demographic groups increased from 1989 to 2004.

The key question raised by this analysis is whether these changes in obstetrics lead to better birth outcomes. There are two schools of thought on this. One view is that many C-sections and inductions are not medically necessary. Thus, by this view, these interventions are doing more harm than good.[4] The alternative view of the high rates of medically induced preterm birth is that, since many medically induced preterm births are done for valid medical reasons, they may be a key factor in preventing fetal and infant mortality. Circumstantial evidence for the latter hypothesis comes from the concurrence of these changes in obstetrics with decreased infant and fetal mortality rates.[5] In the next few chapters, we will examine these competing hypotheses.

Before, we do, however, we need to take care of you.

15 Your Fetus Becomes a Baby

You go to see your doctor the next day. The abdominal pains are about the same. You have barely slept in three days. Your head is aching from the articles you've been reading about late preterm birth and stillbirth and physician-induced demand for C-sections and home birth and spiritual midwifery. You still want what you have always and only wanted, a healthy baby. True, you had imagined what the delivery would be like over and over again. You had wondered how other women did it and whether you would be able to. You worried about the pain and the tears and the bleeding and the episiotomy.

Your doctor examines you. Your cervix is not at all dilated.

She straps a fetal monitor around your belly. The monitor shows that your abdominal pains are, in fact, uterine contractions. They are not strong ones and they are irregular, but they are definitely contractions. You worry. If these are mild contractions, what will the strong ones feel like?

The fetal heart tracing shows that your little fetus has a good heart rate. There is some, but not too much, variability. There are no decelerations after contractions. All good.

You go home again.

The pains become more regular. The contractions are getting stronger. You have some fluid leaking from your vagina. You're not sure if your water has broken or not. You return to the hospital. They examine you again and do some vaginal swabs. Yes, they say, your water has broken. Your doctor recommends an induction of labor to strengthen and regularize the contractions. (You later learn that the American College of Obstetrics and Gynecology might have questioned this recommendation.)[1] You trust your doctor.

They start Pitocin. The labor pains get stronger and stronger until they are almost unbearable. Your doctor suggests epidural anesthesia. You readily accept. Anything to stop this pain. Getting the epidural is physically awkward. As the contractions continue, you have to sit up and bend over while they stick a needle in your back. But the relief is almost instant and amazing.

Labor slows. Now, it is almost like it is happening to someone else. You watch the mysterious tracings on the monitor, listen to the whispers of the doctors and the nurses. Soon, the whispers become a little more urgent, a little more worried. Your doctor tells you that the baby's heart rate is not right. She says it is time to get the baby out with a C-section.

16   A Defense of Modern Obstetrics

Defenders of modern obstetrics point to the measurable improvements in maternal health that have resulted from a proactive, technologically sophisticated, and hospital-based approach to the management of labor and delivery. Those improvements have been dramatic. In 1900, nearly 1 in every 100 women who gave birth would die. Today, death occurs in only 1 in 10,000 deliveries, a 99% reduction in maternal mortality.

These dramatic statistics do not, however, clinch the case for modern obstetrics. They both reveal and conceal some truths. As with every other aspect of pregnancy, labor, and childbirth, even the terminology is contentious.

The term "maternal mortality" used to refer only to death during pregnancy, labor, and delivery. The maternal mortality rate was seen as the best measure of the safety and efficacy of medical care during these events. Then, with the advent of oral contraception in the 1960s and the legalization of abortion in the 1970s, there were new sorts of mortality associated with procreation and with efforts to prevent procreation. Some women died as a result of complications from oral contraceptives. "Maternal mortality" has become "pregnancy-related mortality" since not all pregnant women become mothers. (Of course, abortion-related mortality was a factor in pregnancy-related mortality even before abortion was legal.) And even that doesn't quite cover all of the mortality associated with the health care and disease that is associated with contraception and pregnancy. In 1982, Sachs and colleagues at the Centers for Disease Control suggested a different phrase, "reproductive mortality," to encompass any and all deaths associated with contraception, pregnancy, abortion, or childbirth. They used the concept to analyze trends. Between 1955 and 1975, the overall mortality rate for women 15 through 44 years of age fell by 73%, from 7.8 to 2.1 per 100,000 women.[1] The fall came about because of a few separate but interrelated phenomena. There was a dramatic decline in overall, allcause mortality rates over the three decades. In the 1950s, most of the reproductive mortality in this age group was from complications of pregnancy. In later periods, a higher percentage of mortality was attributable to pregnancy prevention. The use of oral contraceptives, in particular, accounted for a larger and larger percentage of overall mortality. Most of this contraceptive-related mortality was in women over the age of 35.

Oral contraceptives were not available in 1955. By 1965, they caused 14% of all reproductive mortality. By 1982, half of the deaths related to reproductive health were attributable to contraception-related causes and half to complications of childbirth. Since the 1980s, the deaths attributable to both contraception and childbirth have steadily fallen. The proportions remain roughly the same. Here are the raw numbers: In 1975, there were 492 deaths in the United States related to childbirth, 556 related to contraception, and 35 related to induced abortion. The rate of maternal mortality reached its lowest point in 1987. That year, there were 548 deaths related to childbirth for a rate of 0.66 per 10,000 women of reproductive age. Since then, the rate has been rising. In 2007, the rate was 1.27 per 10,000 women. Deaths related to contraception have fallen, probably because oral contraceptives use lower doses of estrogen and because women over 35, the group at highest risk, have shifted to other methods of contraception.

The dramatic improvements in overall reproductive mortality came to an end in the 1980s. For the last thirty years, pregnancy-related mortality in the United States has stayed stubbornly the same, even as the technology of obstetrics has intensified and rates of C-section and labor induction have skyrocketed. This leveling off supports the overall theme of this book, that obstetrics today is focused as much on fetal health as on maternal health. Obstetricians routinely do things—like your C-section—that increase the risks to pregnant women in order to improve the outcomes for babies.

And there have been dramatically better outcomes for babies. Even as preterm birth rates have risen, both infant mortality rates and fetal mortality rates have dropped.

K. S. Joseph offers one of the more powerful theoretical and epidemiological arguments for this point of view.[2] He suggests that modern obstetrics can no longer be evaluated by metrics such as preterm birth rates or even infant mortality. Instead, he suggests that we use new metrics that take into account the new ways that we now assess the health of the fetus. By this approach, the measure of obstetric success should be the survival rate of all living fetuses that attain 20 weeks of gestation. He calls this the "fetus at risk" approach. This approach recognizes that, for women and their doctors, the difference between a fetal death and an infant death is often essentially irrelevant. Once a decision has been made to not terminate pregnancy, the goal is to keep both the pregnant woman and the fetus healthy.

Most of the time, the interests of these two patients are aligned. Sometimes, they are not. Joseph explains the difference between traditional measures of pregnancy outcomes and his new proposal as follows:

Under the traditional model of perinatal death, neonatal deaths occur among infants in the first month after birth and the unborn fetus is not a candidate for neonatal death. However from a broad biological, obstetric and ultimately epidemiologic point of view, a fetus at any gestation is at risk of stillbirth and neonatal death at that gestation. If one considers a woman at 28 weeks gestation with severe preeclampsia and fetal compromise, the risk of stillbirth is easy to conceptualize. The risk of neonatal death is substantial as well and can follow either premature labour or medically indicated delivery....Thus, although neonatal deaths literally occur among infants, fetuses can be considered candidates for neonatal death as well.

With his colleagues, he analyzed pregnancy outcome data in the United States, Canada, and some European countries using this approach.[3] It was not an easy study to do because different countries use different approaches to decide which fetal deaths and which births to report. Joseph and colleagues assessed the total reported rates of infant mortality and of stillbirth in these countries. They then did the same analysis excluding live-born babies under 500 grams and again excluding live-born babies under 1,000 grams. They did this because their theory was that many countries do not report the tiniest babies as live births and that, as a result, their reported infant mortality rates are lower than their actual infant mortality rates. If this theory is correct, then some countries' infant mortality rates seem low because they completely exclude a certain group of babies, those who are born alive at low gestational ages and who then die quickly. In some countries, these are classified as live births and infant deaths. In other countries, apparently, they are classified as stillbirths. By comparing mortality rates after completely excluding these tiny babies, Joseph et al could test their theory about unreported exclusions.

Their results supported their theory. They found wide variation in the reported proportion of live births with a birthweight of less than 500 grams. Reported rates of live birth at under 500 grams were lower than 1 per 10,000 live births in Belgium, Ireland, Latvia, Poland, Portugal, and the Slovak Republic. By contrast, they were 6.1 in England and Wales, 10.8 in Canada, and 16.9 in the United States. Neonatal death rates were correspondingly low in the countries that reported few such live births. When they analyzed the percentage of all reported neonatal deaths that were accounted for babies weighing less than 500 grams, they found similar variations—less than 1% of neonatal deaths in many countries, less than 15% in Europe, and 30% in Canada and the United States. Clearly, in many countries, live-born babies are classified as stillbirths. There is no way to know for certain whether these observed differences in the proportion of live births and stillbirths at extremely low birthweight reflect true differences in those rates between countries. However, the differences are striking, and the countries' policies for reporting live births are known to vary widely and in ways that are consistent with those policies. The most likely explanation is that, in many countries, such deaths simply are not reported or considered in calculations of neonatal mortality rates.

They then made hypothetical calculations of the true neonatal mortality rate in these different countries, assuming that the rate of birth at each gestational age was the same. They found that there was far less variation than there was in reported infant mortality. For example, by this measure, the United States had a lower neonatal mortality rate than the UK, Norway, Denmark, and the Netherlands.

They also found that the countries with the lowest reported rates of infant mortality had the highest reported rates of stillbirth. This also supports the theory that, in some countries, babies born at the borderline of viability who die quickly are categorized as stillbirths rather than as neonatal deaths.

The best measure of overall mortality, then, is one called "perinatal mortality." That is a measure of deaths between 20 weeks of gestation and one month of age after birth. Using this measure, the perinatal mortality rates in most of these countries was quite similar, again suggesting that there are differences in the way different countries classify some births as either a live birth with infant mortality or a stillbirth.

These data do not, of course, validate modern approaches to obstetrics. But, taken together with overall declines in infant mortality in all of these countries, the data suggest that the combination of interventionist obstetrics with a focus on the fetus at risk and the availability of neonatal intensive care for even the tiniest preterm babies have led to a suite of practices that have successfully lowered rates of both fetal and infant mortality. Further, the data suggest that at least part of that success is a result of obstetricians' willingness to induce early delivery if it appears to be the best thing for the fetus at risk. Such a calculus, of course, could only be advantageous in places where neonatal intensive care is readily available, so that the baby born after a preterm induction or C-section can be successfully treated for the problems associated with prematurity. But such care is readily available today in all industrialized countries and, as we show in the next chapter, it has had a profound effect on the mortality rates of preterm infants.

17   Neonatal Intensive Care and Infant Mortality

Neonatal intensive care was developed during the same time period as most of the other changes we have described in this book. It came into existence, in its modern form, in the mid-1960s, during the same years when Liley was pioneering intrauterine transfusions and women were starting to use the pill and Hon was developing intrauterine fetal monitoring and Nadler figured out how to diagnose chromosomal anomalies in the fetus.

Neonatal intensive care was made possible by the development of positive pressure ventilators suitable for premature babies. Such ventilators had been used for adults with respiratory failure since 1952 when they had been pioneered as a treatment for polio.[1] By the late 1950s, many hospitals had intensive care units for critically ill adults.[2]

Mechanical ventilation for babies was developed in Toronto in the mid-1960s. Soon, many large medical centers in the United States had opened neonatal intensive care units (NICUs) in which premature babies with respiratory distress syndrome could be treated and kept alive by positive pressure ventilation. This allowed doctors to save babies who were born preterm and whose lungs were not fully developed. Enabling these babies to breathe soon led to the need for other supportive therapies, including treatment of infections, surgery for congenital anomalies, and innovative ways of providing nutrition.

While first used to treat prematurity, the technology of the NICU made it possible for doctors also to treat term babies with congenital anomalies. Those babies frequently needed complex surgery. Their postoperative care required the same level of support that was needed by premature babies. Throughout the 1960s and 1970s, doctors became adept at treating babies with congenital heart disease, diaphragmatic hernias, myelomeningocele, and other anomalies that had once been considered untreatable and fatal. All of these developments led to rapid and dramatic improvements in infant mortality.

In 1960, the infant mortality rate in the United States was 25 deaths per 1000 live births. Over the next 25 years, it fell by 60%. By 1986, infant mortality was just 10.1 per 1,000 live births.[3] By 2014, it had nearly halved again, to 5.74 per 1,000. The infant mortality rate fell for almost every cause of death, including infections, congenital malformations, prematurity, and sudden infant death syndrome. For babies born at term, the mortality rate fell from 15 to 5 per 1,000, a drop of 67%. For babies born between 32 and 36 weeks of gestation, the drop was even more dramatic— from 75 to 16.5 deaths per 1,000, a drop of 78%. For babies born before 32 weeks, infant mortality rates fell by 63% but remained high at 213 deaths per 1,000 live births.

Premature babies continued to have higher mortality rates than full-term babies. Throughout the 1990s, the rate of medically induced preterm birth rose steadily.[4] The rise likely reflected a belief that the risks of late preterm birth were lower than they actually were. This belief was more or less accurate for babies born at 36 weeks, that is, just one week before term. For such babies, infant mortality rates were quite similar to babies born at term. (As we have seen, however, there are now questions about whether 37 weeks should be considered "term.") As a result, doctors and pregnant women often decided to medically induce delivery at that point if there were any sign of fetal distress. In 2006, infant mortality rates for babies born at 32 to 36 weeks had fallen to 8.2 in 1,000—still four times higher than the rate for babies born at term in 2006, but quite low by historical standards. This improvement may have reinforced some complacency among obstetricians, and some unwarranted optimism among neonatologists, about the safety of medically induced preterm birth.

Was that a mistake? It is difficult to prove one way or the other. Joseph and colleagues analyzed whether the increase in medically induced preterm birth led to an overall increase in infant mortality or serious neonatal morbidity. They found that, over the years from 1995 to 2005 in the United States, stillbirth rates declined, rates of medically induced preterm birth rose, and neonatal mortality rates declined. More important, they found that the decline in neonatal mortality was greater for babies born after a medically induced preterm birth than after a spontaneous preterm birth. It thus appears that, in a world of careful fetal monitoring, judicious use of medically induced delivery, and neonatal intensive care, a proactive approach to obstetrics leads to an overall decline in infant mortality for near-term babies. That is, even though their mortality rate is higher than that of term babies, it is lower than it was before the increase in medically induced deliveries.

That population-level claim cannot, however, justify specific clinical decisions in a given situation; that is, it doesn't indicate whether or not a particular medically induced preterm birth

would be beneficial. But it is probably impossible to study different approaches to delivery situations in a rigorous way. It would
be very difficult to do a prospective randomized trial of different
obstetrical approaches following signs of fetal distress. Instead,
as in our paradigmatic case of the 34-year-old expectant mother,
the doctor and patient make the best decision that they can
under conditions of significant uncertainty, motivated—for the
patient in particular—by fear of a disastrous outcome.

Such dilemmas highlight one of the themes of our analysis,
which is that the very nature of prenatal care has changed dramatically in the recent decades. The next chapter discusses the
profound nature of those changes.

18   The Evolution of Prenatal Care

To summarize our argument thus far: we began with the frustrating mystery of the rising rate of preterm birth in the face of sustained efforts to lower that rate. We showed how those efforts to reduce infant mortality focused first on improving access to prenatal care. We observed that improved access to prenatal care did not seem to work. That is, throughout the 1990s, more pregnant women received prenatal care but preterm birth rates continued to rise. We analyzed changes in the demography of childbearing and the effect that those changes might have had on the rate of preterm birth. Those changes, though dramatic, also did not explain the inexorable rise in prematurity. Instead, the rise in preterm birth is clearly associated with changing obstetrical practices. It is, in that sense, an iatrogenic problem. But it is a peculiar sort of iatrogenic problem in that it is not an unintended, unforeseen, or incidental consequence of medical treatment. Instead, it is a consequence that grows out of a new view of what prenatal care ought to be and do. That new view has evolved over the last half-century, but it has rarely been acknowledged. The essence of the new view is that prenatal care is no longer solely about the health of the pregnant woman. The fetus has become a second patient. We will now try to put together the story of what prenatal care used to be, what it has

become, and the ways in which these changes might paradoxically have led to more, rather than fewer, preterm births.

Prenatal Care in the Early Twentieth Century

One of the best descriptions of prenatal care in the early twentieth century is in a booklet entitled *Prenatal Care* that was
issued in 1913 by the newly formed Children's Bureau of the
United States Department of Labor.[1] (The creation of the Children's Bureau and its early decision to focus on prenatal care as
an appropriate use of the minuscule budget that Congress had
appropriated for its work is a good story, perhaps even a relevant
story, but is beyond the scope of this book.) The prenatal care
booklet was a very practical self-help book designed for pregnant
women and women who were thinking of becoming pregnant.
It was written by Mrs. Max West (Mary Mills West) in a folksy,
down-to-earth style. Mrs. West was good at what she did. Her
books on prenatal care and child rearing would sell more than
60 million copies. The book beautifully illustrates what prenatal
care used to be.

Prenatal Care begins, appropriately enough, by describing the
signs that women should look for in order to determine if they
are pregnant. Mrs. West lists four: (1) cessation of menstruation;
(2) changes in the breasts; (3) morning sickness; and (4) disturbances in urination. In 1913, there were no blood tests or urine
tests or imaging studies that could be done to confirm or rule out
pregnancy. The ultimate confirmatory sign was "quickening," or
the movement of the fetus in the uterus. That usually took place
at around the sixteenth or eighteenth week of pregnancy.

Mrs. West gave commonsense advice about healthy living.
Pregnant women were to drink lots of liquids, eat fruits and

vegetables but not much meat, and consume enough for two people. Prunes and figs were recommended for constipation. Mrs. West recommended an hour or two per day of exercise in the fresh air. There is an extensive discussion of what a pregnant woman should wear. "The ordinary corset should be discarded early in pregnancy...Comfortable well fitting shoes are a first requisite."[2] There are suggestions as to how to design and sew maternity clothes.

The section of the book entitled "Complications of Pregnancy and How to Avoid Them" discusses disturbances of the kidneys, nausea and vomiting, heartburn, varicose veins, hemorrhoids, cramps, and leukorrhea (vaginal discharge). There is a section on toxemia that includes a description of the symptoms ("persistent vomiting, repeated headaches, dizziness, puffiness about the face and hands, blurring of the vision or spots before the eyes, neuralgic pains") as well as advice about how to prevent it ("guard scrupulously against continued constipation, strive to be happy, seek self-control, and do not worry.") If the symptoms persist, the woman is encouraged to call her doctor.

This is followed by a much longer section on "maternal impressions," the name given to the belief that "if the mother is injured in some way or sees another person injured or observes a deformed or defective person that the impression thus made upon her mind will repeat itself in some corresponding defect in the child's body." Mrs. West is skeptical about the power of maternal impressions but is clearly aware that most women at the time believed them to be powerful influences on the outcomes of pregnancy. So she offers three different lines of argument in an effort to debunk as unscientific the belief in maternal impressions.

The first argument she offers is a physiological one. She writes, "So far as is known there is no connection between the mother and the child in the uterus by which nervous impressions can be conveyed...The mother's blood never enters the child, so that even if the blood were able to convey nervous impressions, the fact that the two circulations are separate and distinct makes the direct injury of the child in this way an impossibility." Her second argument is epidemiological, "There are few mothers who have not at some time during their pregnancies had experiences of a disturbing nature of greater or less severity. Accordingly most babies ought to be born 'marked,' if this belief is true. Manifestly this is not the case." Finally, she offers an argument based on developmental biology: "Many women do not realize that they are pregnant until the sixth or eighth week, and do not usually begin to worry about the baleful effects which they hear talked about until pregnancy is well advanced. Investigation has shown that the form of the child is established by the beginning of the third month, therefore disturbing events which occur in the later months plainly can have no effect."

The discussion of maternal impressions ends with a strong exhortation to pregnant women to worry about the things that truly matter rather than the things that do not. "If then (the pregnant woman) lives in such a manner as to establish and conserve her own health, taking plenty of sleep and exercise, eating sensibly of simple food, and in every way striving to take the best possible care of her own body so that the digestive, assimilative, and excretory functions are carried on in the highest degree of efficiency, she can be quite sure that the child will be able thereby to build up for himself a sound and normal body and brain."

She then discusses labor and delivery. Mrs. West assumes that birth will take place at home. There are detailed instructions on what supplies to have on hand for a delivery at home. ("One hundred bichloride of mercury tablets, four ounces powdered boric acid, one bottle of white Vaseline, one pound of castile soap, one quart of grain alcohol, one douche pan, one stiff hand brush, one slop jar or covered enamel bucket, three pottery or agateware basins, one and one-half yards of white table oilcloth, to protect the mattress.") Also, instructions are given on when to call the doctor and the nurse and what to do if the baby is born before the doctor arrives.

The final chapters discuss the care of the baby, the importance of breastfeeding, and the appropriate diet for a nursing mother.

We quote this book at some length for a few reasons. First, Mrs. West was a good writer. She wrote a practical book, packed with information presented in a beautifully accessible style. Second, the book illustrates the approach to prenatal care that was predominant for the first half of the twentieth century. The goal of prenatal care at that time was to improve outcomes for both pregnant women and their babies. The only way to do that was to encourage the pregnant woman to take excellent care of herself, both physically and psychologically. There was no way to assess the health or the well-being of the fetus. Whatever was going on in the womb was unobservable, mysterious, and beyond the scope of medical assessment.

Over the next hundred years, this approach to prenatal care gave way to a new approach whereby the fetus can be observed, assessed, diagnosed, and sometimes even treated while still in the womb. That approach shattered the holistic unity of pregnancy, the idea that mother and fetus were one entity, that the fetus was an indivisible part of the mother, and that the only way to care for the fetus was to envelop it in a healthy, safe mother.

The new view of prenatal care sees Mrs. West's approach as quaint, archaic, and unsophisticated. By this view, the great advances in perinatal care of the second half of the twentieth century that led to dramatic drops in maternal, infant, and fetal mortality have all come about because we have taken a very different approach to prenatal care. We still, of course, encourage women to eat right, think right, and behave properly (no smoking, drinking, eating cheese or sushi, taking drugs, changing cat litter, etc.) but we also rely on doctors to do the proper tests, carefully monitoring many fetal biochemical and physiological parameters. These careful assessments of the fetus sometimes lead to treatments that benefit the baby but are not necessarily beneficial for the mother.

These two views of prenatal care coexist today in a tension that is sometimes cheerful, sometimes bitter. The relative merits of each are difficult to quantify. The older, more holistic approach continues to guide much health policy. The newer, more technological approach guides much of obstetrical practice. The older approach views prenatal care as something a woman does for herself, with gentle and mostly hands-off guidance from her doctor (although a less highly trained professional could easily handle the guidance). The newer approach sees prenatal care as something that a doctor provides for a woman and her fetus. The older approach favors natural childbirth. The newer approach leads to and accepts higher rates of C-section and medical induction of labor, often prior to term. The older approach is one that, if effective, might be associated with fewer preterm births. (We say "might" because the studies of this approach to prenatal care when it was the only approach all had some flaws. Thus, we can only speculate about its effectiveness. Below, we review some studies examining efforts to provide this sort of prenatal care to high-risk women that suggest that it does not have much effect.) The newer approach may increase the rate of preterm birth but also lead to lower rates of fetal and infant mortality.

Assessing Prenatal Care Today

Prenatal care today is a combination of three things. First, it continues to be the old-fashioned, woman-oriented, preventive treatment that was described by Mrs. West a century ago. However, prenatal care now includes an increasing number of techniques of fetal assessment and treatment, pioneered by Liley and Lejeune and refined over the last fifty years. Second, prenatal care uses this information to diagnosis fetal conditions that cannot be treated and to inform parents who may want to consider abortion. Third, information about fetal health can also be used to determine whether the fetus has a condition that would benefit from treatment. Treatment could be in utero fetal surgery, medication designed to treat fetal disease, or obstetrical intervention to deliver the fetus early. These distinct elements of prenatal care have different goals, lead to different outcomes, and require consideration and balancing of different risks and benefits. So prenatal care today has multiple purposes and goals. They sometimes conflict with each other.

The complicated nature of prenatal care today—and the conceptual confusion about the mother-centered and fetus-centered components—is beautifully illustrated by the description of such care on the website of the U.S. Department of Health and Human Services. The site has a page called Women's Health at www.womenshealth.gov. The section on "Pregnancy" begins, "Becoming a mother is one of the most exciting times in a woman's life."

There is an extensive discussion of prenatal care. It starts by explaining the differences between obstetricians, family practice doctors, certified nurse-midwives, and doulas. It explains the advantages and disadvantages of births in hospitals, birthing centers, and at home. It delves into the details of prenatal care, noting that

At your first visit your doctor will perform a full physical exam, take your blood for lab tests, and calculate your due date. Your doctor might also do a breast exam, a pelvic exam to check your uterus (womb), and a cervical exam, including a Pap test. During this first visit, your doctor will ask you lots of questions about your lifestyle, relationships, and health habits. It's important to be honest with your doctor. After the first visit, most prenatal visits will include checking your blood pressure and weight, checking the baby's heart rate, and measuring your abdomen to check your baby's growth. You also will have tests to look for anemia, tests to measure risk of gestational diabetes, and tests to look for harmful infections.[3]

All this is part of traditional prenatal care, that is, prenatal care designed to promote the health of the pregnant woman as the best way to insure a healthy baby. The "baby's heart rate" is the only assessment of the fetus.

Then, the discussion turns to assessments of the health of the fetus. It begins with a recommendation to the pregnant woman that she keep track of her baby's movement and call her doctor if she counts less than 10 movements within two hours.

The website goes on to describe a series of screening tests that might be done to diagnose problems in the fetus. There is a description of the techniques and goals of amniocentesis, biophysical profiling, chorionic villus sampling, first trimester screen, a non-stress test, and an ultrasound examination.

The website then explains that certain pregnancies are classified as high risk, and for those pregnancies doctors may recommend more tests or more frequent visits. As the website elaborates on these tests, we realize that we've left the domain of traditional prenatal care and suddenly but subtly have entered the domain of fetal medicine. None of the tests that are then described were available before the 1960s. All are used to diagnose disease or distress in the fetus. Many remain controversial. As an example, consider the use of ultrasound during pregnancy. Ultrasound first became available for routine clinical use in the 1970s. From the outset, experts debated how and when it should be used.

In 1984, a consensus conference convened by the National Institutes of Health noted that there was no good evidence to show that routine ultrasound was beneficial in low-risk pregnancies. It recommended against routine screening unless and until randomized controlled trials showed some benefit.[4] Studies were done. Between 1987 and 1991, a study sponsored by NIH enrolled 15,000 low-risk women at 109 practice sites throughout the United States. Women were randomly assigned to receive or not receive a routine ultrasound screening exam. The outcome measure was an adverse perinatal outcome, defined as fetal or neonatal death, or moderate/severe problems in the baby. The rates of adverse perinatal outcome were 5% in the screening group and 4.9% in the control group.[5] The authors concluded that routine screening was useless and expensive. They estimated that it would increase annual national expenditures on prenatal care by $1 billion without providing any benefit.

A similar trial in Europe, however, showed that routine screening effectively identified 73% of all major fetal anomalies.[6] Many women whose fetuses were thus identified chose abortion, leading to a lower overall perinatal mortality rate in the group that received ultrasound screening.

These two studies, taken together, suggest the different ways that prenatal screening tests can be used. One is to improve pregnancy outcomes in low-risk pregnancies for the live-born babies, as suggested by the study design of the U.S. ultrasound study. There is not much evidence for the effectiveness of this use. Another is to detect fetal anomalies in order to terminate pregnancy, as suggested by the European study. A third way that prenatal ultrasound can be useful, one that has been both touted and criticized, is simply to satisfy consumer demand.[7] Ultrasound images have become a new form of baby picture.

Even though there has never been a randomized trial that showed routine ultrasound screening in low-risk pregnancies to be beneficial, its use has steadily increased. Between the mid-1990s and the mid-2000s, the average number of ultrasound examinations done in each pregnancy nearly doubled, to about 2.7 ultrasounds per pregnancy.[8]

As the technology has evolved, another clinical use for ultrasound has emerged. Fetal anomalies can be identified in order to offer in utero surgery or to plan postnatal interventions.[9] The most dramatic example of this is in the current approach to prenatal diagnosis and treatment of myelomeningocele (MMC), also known as spina bifida. The story of different approaches to the diagnosis and treatment of MMC is illustrative of the changes that have occurred in the way we think about the fetus as a patient.

Maternal-Fetal Surgery for Congenital Anomalies

Myelomeningocele (MMC) is the most common severe congenital anomaly of the central nervous system.[10,11] Annually, about 1500 babies are born with MMC in the United States. Approximately two-thirds of pregnant women who receive an early diagnosis of fetal MMC elect to terminate the pregnancy.[12] Thus, the prevalence of MMC in fetuses is likely at least twice as high as the birth prevalence.

MMC causes a variety of neurologic problems. The most prominent is paralysis below the level of the MMC lesion. Many babies with MMC have club feet. Almost all babies with MMC have malformations of the brain that cause hydrocephalus. Most children have some cognitive or learning problems.

Approximately 14% of infants born with MMC die within the first five years of life. Mortality rates are twice that high for patients with the Arnold-Chiari malformation than for others. However, most people with MMC live well into adulthood.[13]

There have been four approaches to diagnose and treat MMC. One is primary prevention through prenatal folate supplementation. A second is prenatal diagnosis and the termination of pregnancy. The third approach is prenatal in utero surgery. Finally, doctors can repair the MMC lesion postnatally.

In 1980, Smithells and colleagues suggested that periconceptional supplementation with multivitamins could reduce the risk of MMC.[14] While the mechanism is not known, current hypotheses suggest that MMC and other neural tube defects may be caused either by a folate deficiency or an abnormal metabolic pathway that requires folate.[15] Folate supplementation has reduced the prevalence of MMC. In England and Wales, it has led to a decline from 3.6 cases per 1000 live births to 0.3 cases, making it one of the major public health successes of the twentieth century.[16]

Prenatal diagnosis of MMC has evolved over the last four decades. In the 1970s, doctors began testing serum alpha fetoprotein (AFP) levels in pregnant women as a screening test for MMC.[17] Elevated AFP levels indicate an increased risk of MMC. Such screening allowed the detection of 65% to 83% of pregnancies in which the fetus had MMC.[18,19]

Fetal ultrasound was introduced as a technique to diagnose MMC in 1975.[20] Ultrasound screenings are now standard and can conclusively diagnose fetal MMC at rates that approach 100% in the first trimester.[21] Once a diagnosis of fetal MMC is confirmed, the severity of the defect can be analyzed based on ultrafast MRI images.[22]

MMC is not a lethal anomaly. Most babies born with MMC survive. However, they survive with the lifelong problems noted above—hydrocephalus, paraplegia, and cognitive deficits. Until the late 1990s, the only intervention that was available to women whose fetus was diagnosed with MMC was to terminate the pregnancy. That changed with the development of in utero, maternal-fetal surgery to repair the spinal lesion after a prenatal diagnosis of MMC.[23] In the late 1990s and early 2000s, such surgery was developed in a few tertiary care centers but it was unclear whether it was actually beneficial. Preliminary clinical studies suggested that babies born after in utero surgery had better motor function and were less likely to require ventriculoperitoneal shunts.[24,25] There was some evidence of increased cognitive function at two years of age. But such surgery was complex and risky. It had to be performed late in the second trimester and sometimes led to premature labor and the birth of an extremely premature baby. It was unclear whether outcomes were, in fact, better for the babies born after such surgery.

The debates mirrored those that had taken place over intrauterine transfusion for EBF decades before. The key question was whether there were some pregnancies in which the risks outweighed the benefits.

As a result of the ongoing controversy about the indication for, and outcomes after, maternal-fetal surgery, three leading centers proposed a prospective randomized controlled trial.

The trial was complicated to carry out, both technically and ethically.

Between 2003 and 2010, the Children's Hospital of Philadelphia, Vanderbilt University Medical Center, and the University of California at San Francisco designed and conducted a study called the Management of Myelomeningocele Study (MOMS). The MOMS was a prospective, randomized trial designed to determine whether maternal-fetal surgery led to decreased brain herniation, increased extremity function, and decreased hydrocephalus and need for shunting. The study also analyzed whether such surgery led to increased preterm birth, increased infant mortality, or increased obstetrical complications for the pregnant woman.[26]

The MOMS showed that surgery was beneficial. The study compared two groups on the basis of a composite outcome of fetal or neonatal death or the need for placement of a cerebrospinal fluid shunt by the age of 12 months. The babies in the group that received treatment had a lower percentage of poor outcomes than those in the control group (68% v. 98%), and the trial provided highly statistically significant evidence that this difference did not occur by chance ($P < 0.001$). With regard to neurodevelopmental outcome at 30 months of age, babies in the treatment group also did better. However, prenatal surgery was indeed associated with specific risks for the mother and the fetus: increased risks of preterm delivery, uterine rupture at the surgical site at the time of delivery, and placental abruption.

The MOMS is a striking example of a prenatal intervention that clearly increases the risk of preterm birth, increases health risks to the pregnant woman, yet improves the outcome for the baby. It forces pregnant women, their doctors, and policy makers to decide how fetal interests (and the related interests of the child that the fetus will become) should be weighed against the interests of the pregnant woman.

Such surgery is ethically and medically controversial.[27] It is also just the tip of the iceberg of such dilemmas. Consider that, in the MOMS, surgery was done when the fetus was between 20 and 25 weeks of gestation. However, animal studies and human experience have suggested that if the surgery were initiated earlier, there could be even greater benefit to the baby.[28] The danger in this, of course, is the risk of premature delivery, which gets more dangerous with younger fetal ages. Proceeding too early could injure the fetus, cause intrauterine fetal death, or lead to delivery prior to viability. It would also likely increase the risk of complications related to prematurity, offsetting the benefit from reduced MMC symptoms.[29] Adzick suggests that the solution might lie in developing less invasive surgical methods that "may not only minimize preterm labor and delivery, but may also permit prenatal coverage of the lesion much earlier in gestation."[30]

Myelomeningocele provides an illustrative example of the way prenatal care fulfills multiple functions. Prenatal care that recommends early maternal supplementation with folates (a month preconception and during the first trimester) can reduce the risk. Prenatal care can establish a fetal diagnosis in order to enable termination of pregnancy, but it can also establish a fetal diagnosis to inform an intervention. The diagnosis can also help guide decisions about labor and delivery. Each of these responses to a diagnosis would have a very different effect on infant mortality and the rate of preterm birth. Elective termination of pregnancies in cases of congenital anomalies would lower the rate of both infant mortality and preterm birth.[31] In utero surgery or elective preterm delivery might increase the rate of both.[32]

These possibilities illustrate the different goals of prenatal care. They show how the use of evidence-based medicine to decide what technologies should or should not be routinely employed in prenatal care, as well as in labor and delivery, require consideration of trade-offs between fetal health, maternal health, and the health and well-being of newborns. A similar debate surrounds the use of intrauterine fetal monitoring during labor.

As with many of the new technologies of obstetrics, the technology for such intrauterine fetal monitoring had been developed by the late 1950s and was introduced, experimentally, into clinical practice in the 1960s.[33] Hon and colleagues suggested that heart rate decelerations in a fetus were a sign of distress and an indication for an induced early delivery.[34] Some studies seemed to show that such monitoring was effective in preventing perinatal mortality.[35] Others did not.[36] The debate about the efficacy of intrauterine monitoring would rage for decades. A 2013 meta-analysis of dozens of studies showed that fetal monitoring led to fewer cases of neonatal seizures, no differences in mortality or cerebral palsy, and an increase in C-sections and instrumental vaginal deliveries. The authors concluded that there were no clear benefits.[37]

In the meantime, as with ultrasound, clinicians make their own decisions about when these technologies should or should not be used.[38,39] Today, most obstetricians monitor fetal heart rates in most deliveries even though it is not clear that it leads to better outcomes. Devoe acknowledges that, beneficial or not, "the overwhelming majority of laboring patients will continue to receive EFM," and that, rather than trying to decrease the use of such technology, obstetricians should simply try to use it more cautiously.[40]

The debates about intrauterine monitoring, routine ultrasound, and in utero surgery are all examples of debates about the goals of prenatal care and about the best way to take care of fetuses, babies, and pregnant women. In such debates, the data only get us so far. In the end, decisions reflect not just science but also how people make decisions in the face of uncertainty and an emotionally charged situation, how technology shapes those choices, and how policy makers allocate resources so as to promote or discourage certain ways of thinking and acting in response to the challenges.

19   International Comparisons

The conventional wisdom about international comparisons of birth outcomes is that the United States has a much higher rate of infant mortality and preterm birth than most other industrialized countries. Furthermore, the gaps between these rates in the United States and those in other countries seems to be widening. U.S. rates of C-section delivery are also higher than in most other countries.

A 2012 report by the Congressional Research Service, for example, noted that the infant mortality rate in the United States is concerning to policy makers because it is nearly 50% higher than the rate in Europe.[1] Similarly, a 2009 report from the CDC noted that, in 2005, the United States ranked 30th in the world in infant mortality, behind most European countries, Canada, Australia, New Zealand, Hong Kong, Singapore, Japan, and Israel.[2] The authors attribute our higher infant mortality rate to our higher rate of preterm birth, dismiss the claim that this higher rate is merely a reporting artifact, and suggest that the only way we can move up in the international rankings is to lower our rate of preterm birth. They don't say how we could do that.

Studies such as the one by Joseph and colleagues cited in chapter 16 question this conventional wisdom about international differences. They note that there are consistent and documented reporting differences between countries that account for some of the differences in rates of preterm birth and infant mortality. They also note that differences in access to abortion may influence the number of babies born with life-threatening congenital anomalies.

Differences in the recording of live births are only part of the problem. Another missing piece in these comparisons is the rate of fetal death. If, as we suggest, the "fetus at risk" approach is the preferable approach for comparing the efficacy of perinatal health care systems, then the analysis must include not just rates of stillbirth, preterm birth, and infant mortality. It must also examine the rate of prenatal diagnosis of congenital anomalies, the rates of abortion for such anomalies, and the survival rates for live-born babies with such anomalies. The discussion of myelomeningocele in the preceding chapter suggests the ways that prenatal diagnosis and fetal interventions may change the way doctors and parents think about prenatally diagnosed anomalies.

Many studies of infant mortality focus on preterm birth as the primary risk factor for infant mortality. Fewer studies examine the contribution of congenital anomalies, another leading cause of infant deaths. This can lead to mistaken assumptions about the sorts of interventions that might lower infant mortality. Preterm birth is seen as preventable. Congenital anomalies are not. But neither perception is quite accurate.

The assumption that preterm birth is preventable is not borne out by the facts. As we will show in the next chapter, efforts to reduce preterm birth by improving the quality and availability of prenatal care have not been very successful.

Births of babies with congenital anomalies, by contrast, are eminently preventable. To do so, however, requires excellent prenatal diagnosis and the availability of abortion.

Many countries track congenital anomalies. Europe has an international registry of congenital anomalies, EUROCAT, which records live births, fetal deaths after 20 weeks of gestation, and terminations of pregnancy for fetal anomalies (TOPFA).[3] Between 2003 and 2007, in 22 European countries, the total prevalence of major congenital anomalies was 23.9 per 1,000 pregnancies (at 20 weeks of age.) Of these, 80% resulted in a live birth. Two percent were stillbirths after 20 weeks of gestation. In 17.6% of cases, pregnancy was terminated as a result of the diagnosis of a congenital anomaly. No similar statistics are available for the United States so it is hard to compare outcomes. Studies show that the rate of abortion for congenital anomalies is lower in the United States than in much of Europe.[4] This probably reflects both religious or cultural attitudes and the fact that abortion is often not covered by health insurance. This could lead to higher rates of congenital anomalies among live births and higher infant mortality rates.

International comparisons, then, reflect differences in the way countries define live birth and in the comprehensiveness of the reporting of live births even by their own definitions. Those comparisons may also reflect differences in the prevalence of congenital anomalies, the rate at which those congenital anomalies are diagnosed prenatally, and the percentage of pregnancies with congenital anomalies that end in abortion. Any truly accurate international comparisons would have to account for all these factors, and none of the present comparisons do so. Thus international comparisons of infant mortality rates are likely to overestimate the differences between the United States and other countries. The situation here might not be as bad as some such comparisons suggest. The only way to be sure would be to have in place comprehensive and standardized public health reporting systems that kept accurate records of pregnancies, stillbirths, prenatally diagnosed congenital anomalies, induced and spontaneous abortions, live births, and infant deaths. Such systems do not now exist are unlikely to exist in the future. All we can do with existing data is try to draw accurate inferences. These suggest that many of the differences that are often highlighted in international comparisons of perinatal and infant mortality may be based on faulty assumptions about the comparability of the data.

In the 1970s and 1980s, experts were convinced that better prenatal care would lower the rate of preterm birth. Studies showed significant relationships between infant mortality and the lack of prenatal care. These studies, as noted in chapter 1, led the Institute of Medicine to conclude that "prenatal care reduces low birthweight and that the effect is greatest among high-risk women. This finding is strong enough to support a broad national commitment to ensuring that all pregnant women, especially those at socioeconomic or medical risk, receive high quality prenatal care."

The solution to this important problem seemed attractively simple. Increased access to prenatal care would allow all pregnant women to see doctors, have their blood pressure monitored, receive nutritional counseling, get immunized, and stop smoking. It would allow these women and their doctors to plan a delivery in the appropriate setting. Surely, with such a plan, more babies would be born at term, infant mortality rates would drop, and costs would be reduced.

As noted earlier, such arguments convinced lawmakers to significantly expand the Medicaid program so that more women would be eligible for more comprehensive and timely prenatal care. These Medicaid expansions were passed into law in the late 1980s.

Over the next decade, researchers analyzed the effect of the Medicaid expansion on preterm birth. The results were disheartening. In 2001, researchers from the Urban Institute in Washington, DC, published a comprehensive analysis of the effect of the expansions in the Medicaid program. They examined data on over 8 million births, comparing births between 1980 and 1986 to those between 1986 and 1993. They were particularly interested in whether poor women received more prenatal care and whether those women had fewer low birthweight babies.

The researchers showed that, although more women enrolled in prenatal care early in pregnancy and received comprehensive prenatal care throughout pregnancy, there was no decrease in the rate of low birthweight birth. They concluded, "The expansions in Medicaid lead to significant improvements in prenatal care utilization among women of low socioeconomic status. The emerging lesson from the Medicaid expansions, however, is that increased access to primary care is not adequate if the goal is to narrow the gap in newborn health between poor and non-poor populations."[1] Prenatal care was not working the way it had been predicted to work.

Other studies similarly found no effect on birth outcomes. Ray and colleagues studied the effect of Medicaid expansions in Tennessee. They concluded, "In Tennessee, the Medicaid expansions materially increased enrollment and use of prenatal care among high-risk women, but did not reduce the likelihood of preterm birth."[2] Kaestner found little effect of the Medicaid expansions on birth outcomes.[3]

Not all studies were so bleak. Vintzileos and colleagues studied outcomes in all 10 million singleton live births in the United

States between 1995 and 1997.[4] They compared women who received no prenatal care with those who received any prenatal care. They showed that, for pregnant women with no prenatal care, fetal and neonatal death rates were four to five times higher than for mothers with some prenatal care. The group with no prenatal care, however, was extremely small. Of the 10 million pregnant women, only 118,000, or a little over 1%, received no prenatal care. One interpretation of these results was that prenatal care had some benefit, but more prenatal care was not much better than less. Another interpretation was that prenatal care was just a "marker" for other characteristics of mothers that were associated with better birth outcomes. Women who sought prenatal care were more likely to have bigger babies and more full-term babies for reasons unrelated to the prenatal care itself.

Researchers and practitioners have tried to unbundle the components of prenatal care so that they can evaluate the efficacy of different components for carefully defined high-risk populations of pregnant women. In doing so, they tried to figure out which particular pieces of prenatal care might prove particularly efficacious and which might be less so. They developed new and innovative ways to deliver even better and more comprehensive prenatal care. Over the last few decades, these efforts led to eight different prospective randomized trials of different combinations of prenatal interventions. The interventions included better social support, consultation with expert nutritionists, smoking cessation programs, stress reduction programs, subsidized transportation to clinics, and comprehensive screening for vaginal and cervical infections. The goal of these studies was to come up with the absolute ideal comprehensive prenatal care for the women at highest risk for bad outcomes. In short, they tried to both define a new evidence-based approach to prenatal care and, if they could show that it worked, advocate that such high-intensity prenatal care become the standard of care for high-risk pregnancies. Note that these enhancements to prenatal care all focused on the health and support of the mother.

The results of these eight trials were summarized in a meta-analysis published in 1999. In all, the trials enrolled nearly 10,000 pregnant women. Women who were offered psychological counseling, nutritional counseling, transportation to clinic, social support, comprehensive medical screening, and state-of-the-art obstetric services were compared with women who were offered "standard" prenatal care. The conclusions were unambiguous and bleak: "Although observational and quasi-experimental studies have produced a large volume of circumstantial evidence supporting the notion that comprehensive, multicomponent prenatal care prevents low birthweight, studies employing rigorous investigative methods have consistently failed to confirm the efficacy of this intervention strategy."[5]

Lu and colleagues came to similar conclusions.[6] They "reviewed original research, systematic reviews, meta-analyses and commentaries for evidence of effectiveness of the three core components of prenatal care—risk assessment, health promotion and medical and psychosocial interventions—for preventing the two constituents of LBW: preterm birth and intrauterine growth restriction (IUGR)." They found that only two components of prenatal care—smoking cessation programs and antenatal corticosteroid therapy—reduced the rate of preterm delivery. Many other interventions, including bed rest, hydration, sedation, cervical cerclage, progesterone supplementation, antibiotic treatment, psychosocial support, tocolysis (the use of medication to suppress premature labor), and home visitation, yielded insufficient evidence to show efficacy. The researchers

concluded pessimistically, "Neither preterm birth nor intrauterine growth retardation can be effectively prevented by prenatal
care in its present form. Preventing LBW will require reconcep-
tualization of prenatal care as part of a longitudinally and con-
textually integrated strategy to promote optimal development
of women's reproductive health not only during pregnancy, but
over the life course."

Such studies were disturbing not only because they upended
some deeply held beliefs about the efficacy of prenatal care but
also because they raised disturbing concerns about the claims
that universal access to high-quality prenatal care would be cost-
effective. That, also, was called into question. Huntington and
Connell showed that most studies of the cost-effectiveness of
prenatal care had multiple methodological flaws.[7] In particular,
they noted self-selection bias, widely varying and unsupported
estimates of the effectiveness of prenatal care in reducing low
birthweight, underestimates of the cost of comprehensive prenatal care, and oversimplification of the relationship between
changes in low birthweight and actual cost savings. As a result,
they concluded, "The current public perception of prenatal
care oversimplifies the difficulties of delivering prenatal care to
women who do not now receive it, overestimates the benefits of
prenatal care, and contributes to the medicalization of complex
social problems."

Where did all this leave us? In 1980, the infant mortality rate
in the United States was nearly 12.6 per 1,000. Today it is 5.7.
These numbers, while striking, actually underestimate the overall improvements in survival rates for babies. A 2004 report from
the National Center for Health Statistics gives a better picture of
how widespread the improvements have been. That report notes
improvements not just in the rate of infant mortality (death

before one year of age) but also in the rates of neonatal mortality (death before 28 days of age), and late fetal mortality (death in utero after 20 weeks of gestation). They summarize these gains as follows:

[From] 1990 to 2001, the IMR (infant mortality rate) declined 26 percent (from 9.2 to 6.8 per 1,000) for an average decrease of 3 percent per year. Between 1990 and 2001 the neonatal mortality rate declined from 5.8 to 4.5 per 1,000 (down 22 percent). Between 1990 and 2001, the late fetal mortality rate declined fairly steadily, by 23 percent, from 4.3 to 3.3 per 1,000. Although the pace of decline has slowed somewhat since the mid-1990s, significant declines in late fetal mortality and infant mortality have been observed through 2001 despite substantial increases in preterm and low birthweight risk, two important predictors of perinatal health.[8]

Since 2001, outcomes have continued to improve. In 2013, the infant mortality rate in the United States was 5.96 per 1,000, a drop of another 12% since 2001.[9] If this trend continues, our infant mortality rate will be reduced to 4.5 per 1,000 live births by the year 2020.[10]

The paradox, then, is that pregnant women are getting more prenatal care than ever, they are having more preterm births than ever, many of these preterm births are the result of prenatal assessments and obstetrical decisions, and the rate of infant mortality continues to fall.

Since 2006 we have also observed a slow but steady fall in the rate of preterm birth. It peaked in 2006 at a rate of 12.8% of live births. By 2012 it had fallen to 11.5%, a drop of 10%. There are many possible explanations for the recent drop. One is that doctors are doing fewer medically induced preterm deliveries. This is clearly part of the explanation. As a result of efforts by both the March of Dimes and the American College of Obstetrics and Gynecology, the rate of preterm C-sections has dropped. The rate of cesarean delivery for all U.S. births delivered at less than

39 weeks peaked in 2009 at 38.3% and declined in every subsequent year (see figure 5.1), reaching 37.5% in 2012. The drop has been most dramatic at 38 weeks, where the rate has fallen from 34.7 in 2009 to 32.2.[11]

There are other possible explanations for the fall in preterm births. One of the most interesting was put forward by Been and colleagues.[12] They analyzed the effects of smoking bans on the rate of preterm birth. They reviewed eleven different studies from North America and Europe and showed that bans on smoking in public places reduced preterm birth rates by about 10%. This effect was seen in the United States, the United Kingdom, Canada, Ireland, Belgium, and Norway.

It is likely that the drop in preterm birth rates reflects both changes in obstetrics and changes in public health policies, including smoking bans. Both are good for pregnant women and babies. Further reductions might be seen if we could lower the rates of smoking, obesity, and diabetes among pregnant women. It is hard to know, from this data, what the ideal rate of preterm birth ought to be in order to achieve the lowest possible rate of perinatal mortality. Clearly, some medically induced preterm births prevent fetal mortality. Others may increase neonatal mortality. Careful analysis of the indications for medically induced preterm delivery and the outcomes may allow further improvements in perinatal outcomes.

21 Conclusions

We began this inquiry with some speculation about the reasons for the high rate of preterm birth in the United States. We examined the ways in which it might be correlated both with the changing demographics of childbearing and with changes in obstetrics over the last forty years. We hypothesized that these two factors might be linked in that changing obstetrical practices may have been a response to the increasing number of high-risk pregnancies in the United States and that many of those pregnancies were high risk precisely because the average age at childbearing had risen rapidly over these years.

We found that some of our initial hypotheses were true and others were not. Preterm birth rates do not seem to be tightly correlated with changes in the demographics of childbearing. Instead, the complexity of those demographic shifts lead to offsetting influences on preterm birth rates. More childbearing among older women may have led to increased rates of preterm birth. More childbearing among immigrant women may have led to lower rates of preterm birth.

Instead, the only robust association we found was between the rising rate of preterm birth and the rising rate of medical induction of birth. Simply put, we have more preterm births because doctors are choosing to induce delivery before term more often. These preterm inductions are not solely or even primarily in pregnancies that can be classified as high risk. They occur for pregnancies that are high risk, low risk, or of intermediate risk.

The biggest surprise in our analysis was that this shift in obstetrical practices toward a more interventionist approach seems to be associated with improved outcomes for babies. Over the years in which the rate of medically induced preterm birth rates was steadily rising, the rate of both fetal death and neonatal death was steadily falling. The obstetrical choices to induce preterm delivery seem to have had beneficial effects.

This is not to say that there are no risks to a baby from being born prematurely. Extreme prematurity, meaning birth before 32 weeks of gestation, is and has always been associated with high mortality rates. But the analysis in this book has not focused on extreme prematurity. We were more concerned with things that have been changing and there has been no rise—or fall—in rate of extreme prematurity over the last few decades.

The rise in medically induced preterm delivery and the fall in fetal and infant mortality suggest that our way of thinking about the associations between prenatal care, preterm birth, and infant mortality may be mired in outdated or erroneous assumptions about the significance of prenatal care and preterm birth rates for the health of babies. Those old assumptions are that the primary cause of infant mortality is preterm birth and that preterm birth rates can be lowered by providing all women with high-quality prenatal care. The facts are that more women get high-quality prenatal care, preterm birth rates remain stubbornly high, and perinatal mortality continues to fall. Why does all of this matter?

The conclusions drawn from connections between the various measures of the efficacy of prenatal care and obstetrics must consider epidemiological, medical, or social realities. In this brief book, we have tried to suggest some of the ways in which oversimplification of those relationships leads to erroneous conclusions about what is right and what is wrong with the way we care for pregnant women and deliver babies today.

Medical advances have changed the way doctors make decisions about the care of pregnant women and their fetuses. Better prenatal diagnosis, more sensitive fetal monitoring, and widely available neonatal intensive care have changed the implications of the clinical decisions that doctors and pregnant women make. Changes in prenatal care allow more accurate diagnosis of fetal diseases, fetal anomalies, and fetal distress. Such diagnoses often, appropriately, lead doctors to intervene by inducing a preterm delivery. Such interventions often prevent fetal death without increasing infant mortality.

Such changes demand a reevaluation of the conventional wisdom of the 1970s and 1980s that formed the basis for public health and health policy programs over the ensuing three decades. That conventional wisdom was based on data that were collected and analyzed at a time when prenatal and neonatal care were very different than they are today. Current paradigms for evaluating the goals and effectiveness of prenatal care, based on such outdated epidemiology, need to be fundamentally revised. Higher rates of preterm birth clearly are not leading to higher rates of infant mortality. On the contrary, medically induced preterm birth may be essential for lower rates of both fetal and infant mortality.

Evaluated by the "fetus at risk" measures, our current approaches to perinatal health care may be more successful than they sometimes appear, both in terms of trends over time and in terms of contemporaneous international comparisons. We in the United States may be getting better in ways that are not reflected in the traditional measures or perinatal outcomes and other countries may not be as good as their reported outcomes suggest.

Such a revision in our ways of thinking about perinatal health care would require us to upend deeply held beliefs about the nature of pregnancy, the nature of prenatal care, the meaning of preterm birth, the cost-effectiveness of various approaches, the goals we seek to achieve, the measures we use to assess our success, and the public policies we should support.

Whatever one may hold dear in this domain—and, clearly, there are many different ways to think about right and wrong ways of having sex and having babies—it is evident that the ways we get pregnant, prevent pregnancy, and care for pregnant women today differ enormously from the ways we did those things fifty years ago. There are more ways to prevent conception, more ways to induce fertility, greater societal tolerance for wider varieties of behavior in these domains, and a consequent turmoil of moral standards, laws, public policies, and social judgments about what is permissible, impermissible, tolerable, admirable, or immoral. Over the last few decades, we have introduced technologies such as amniocentesis, fetal ultrasonography, karyotyping, intrauterine fetal surgery, in vitro fertilization, fertility drugs, the pill, the morning-after pill, the abortion pill, gestational surrogacy, and selective fetal reduction. Through these technologies, we have greatly expanded the range of reproductive options, so that more people can have healthy babies of their own than ever before and they can have them when they want to have them.

Expansion of the range of available reproductive options comes at a cost. Less natural approaches to pregnancy are usually associated with higher economic costs and greater physical risks to pregnant women, to their fetuses, and to babies. We have bought greater reproductive freedom and better outcomes for both pregnant women and babies by developing a more technological and more highly medicalized approach to pregnancy. Critics of modern obstetrics point out that something is clearly lost when this approach is adopted. We suggest that something is gained as well.

The gains have been gains in reproductive freedoms. Women (and men) today can choose, in ways they never could before, when and how to have babies. They can do so with more confidence than was ever before possible that they will be able to have a baby and that they will likely have a healthy baby. They can make reproductive choices that reflect their values and that are consistent with their life goals.

Of course, there are still no guarantees that every woman will be able to have a healthy baby and have that baby when and how she chooses. But her chances doing so are higher now than they have ever been. This is no small achievement. But it is not usually perceived as an achievement. Instead, traditional measures of success in reproductive health care often focus on outcomes that no longer seem to be the most relevant outcomes.

For forty years, we have focused on increasing rates of C-sections and preterm births as failures to be overcome. We suggest that these measures may overlook other important aspects of perinatal health. Perhaps a better measure would combine an analysis of perinatal mortality, using the "fetus at risk" as the starting point. The goal, then, would be to increase survival among all fetuses that attain 20 weeks of gestation. Such a measure would examine the effects of interventions on fetal mortality as well as on infant mortality.

We might also need to add a factor that reflects the ability of the reproductive health care system to help people achieve their personal goals with regard to pregnancy and childbearing. Did those people who wanted to have children succeed in having children? Did they have them when they wanted to have them? Did the biotechnology associated with reproductive endocrinology, obstetrics, prenatal care, perinatal care, and neonatal care lead to an outcome that those individuals would deem a success? Measures like these could be evaluated over time to see if we are improving. They could be used to compare the success of different health care systems. Compared to the more narrow focus on preterm birth rates and infant mortality, this approach might lead to new ways to evaluate both the successes and the shortcomings of our modern way of having babies.

Notes

Chapter 1

1. Zeitlin J, Szamotulska K, Drewniak N, et al. Preterm birth time trends in Europe: a study of 19 countries. *BJOG* 2013;120:1256–1265.

2. Blencowe H, Cousens S, Oestergaard MZ, et al. National, regional, and worldwide estimates of preterm birth rates in the year 2010 with time trends since 1990 for selected countries: a systematic analysis and implications. *Lancet* 2012;379:2162–2172.

3. Hamilton BE, Martin JA, Ventura SJ. Births: Preliminary data for 2012. National vital statistics reports; vol 62 no 3. Hyattsville, MD: National Center for Health Statistics; 2013.

4. MacDorman MF, Hoyert DL, Matthews DJ. Recent declines in infant mortality in the United States, 2005–2011. NCHS data brief no 120. Hyattsville, MD: National Center for Health Statistics; 2013. http://www.cdc.gov/nchs/data/databriefs/db120.htm. Accessed May 31, 2014.

5. Martin JA, Osterman MJK, Sutton PD. Are preterm births on the decline in the United States? Recent data from the national vital statistics system. NCHS data brief no 39. Hyattsville, MD: National Center for Health Statistics; 2010. http://www.cdc.gov/nchs/data/databriefs/db39.pdf. Accessed February 17, 2015.

6. Woolhandler S, Himmelstein DU. Militarism and mortality: an international analysis of arms spending and infant death rates. *Lancet* 1985;1(8442):1375–1378.

7. Cutler D, Miller G. The role of public health improvements in health advances: the twentieth-century United States. *Demography* 2005;42:1–22.

8. Goldenberg RL, Culhane JF, Iams JD, Romero R. Epidemiology and causes of preterm birth. *Lancet.* 2008;371(9605):75–84. doi:10.1016/S0140-6736(08)60074-4.

9. Institute of Medicine. *Preventing Low Birthweight.* Washington, DC: National Academies Press; 1985. http://books.nap.edu/openbook.php?record_id=511&page=2. Accessed February 17, 2015.

10. Quick JD, Greenlick MR, Roghmann KJ. Prenatal care and pregnancy outcome in an HMO and general population: a multivariate cohort analysis. *Am J Public Health* 1981;71:381–390.

11. Gortmaker SL. The effects of prenatal care upon the health of the newborn. *Am J Public Health* 1979;69:653–660.

12. Senator Lawton Childs, quoted in: Sardell A. Child health policy in the US: the paradox of consensus. *J Health Polit Policy Law* 1990;15:271–304.

13. Loranger L, Lipson D. *The Medicaid Expansions for Pregnant Women and Children.* Washington, DC: The Alpha Center; 1995.

14. Hamilton BE, Minino AM, Martin JA, Kochanek KD, Strobino DM, Guyer B. Annual summary of vital statistics: 2005. *Pediatrics* 2007;119:345–360. http://pediatrics.aappublications.org/cgi/content/full/119/2/345. Accessed February 17, 2015.

15. Centers for Disease Control and Prevention. Infant mortality and low birth weight among Black and White infants—United States, 1980–2000. *MMWR* 2002;51(27):589–592.

16. Institute of Medicine. *Preterm Birth: Causes, Consequences and Prevention.* Washington, DC: National Academies Press; 2007. http://books.nap.edu/openbook.php?record_id=11622&page=2. Accessed February 17, 2015.

17. Surgeon General's Conference on the Prevention of Preterm Birth. http://www.nichd.nih.gov/about/meetings/2008/sg_pretermbirth/ pages/background.aspx. Accessed February 17, 2015.

18. Harris G. Infant deaths drop in the U.S., but the rate is still high. *New York Times*. October 15, 2008. http://www.nytimes.com/2008/ 10/16/health/16infant.html?_r=1& Accessed February 17, 2015.

19. World Health Organization. Country data and rankings for preterm birth data.http://www.who.int/pmnch/media/news/2012/201204_born toosoon_countryranking.pdf. Accessed February 17, 2015.

20. Green J. U.S. has second worst newborn death rate in modern world, report says. CNN.com. May 10, 2006. http://www.cnn.com/2006/ HEALTH/parenting/05/08/mothers.index/. Accessed February 17, 2015.

21. West M. *Prenatal Care*. Washington, DC: U.S. Dept of Labor Children's Bureau; 1913. http://mchlibrary.info/history/chbu/2265-1913 .PDF. Accessed February 17, 2015.

22. Wilson JL, Long SB, Howard PJ. Respiration of premature infants: response to variations of oxygen and to increased carbon dioxide in inspired air. *Am J Dis Child* 1942;63:1080–1085.

23. Hon EH. Electronic evaluation of the fetal heart rate, VI: fetal distress—a working hypothesis. *Am J Obstet Gynecol* 1962;83:333–353.

24. Watson JD, Crick FH. Molecular structure of nucleic acids: a structure for deoxyribose nucleic acid. *Nature* 1953;171(4356):737–738.

25. Kennedy D. *Birth Control in America: The Career of Margaret Sanger*. New Haven, CT: Yale University Press; 1971:263.

26. Paul VI. *Humanae Vitae*. Encyclical letter on the regulation of birth. http://www.vatican.va/holy_father/paul_vi/encyclicals/documents/ hf_p-vi_enc_25071968_humanae-vitae_en.html. Accessed February 17, 2015.

27. Peller AJ, Westgate MN, Holmes LB. Trends in congenital malformations, 1974–1999: effect of prenatal diagnosis and elective termination. *Obstet Gynecol* 2004;104(5 Pt 1):957–964.

Chapter 2

1. Elton C. American women: birthing babies at home. *Time*. October 4, 2010. http://content.time.com/time/magazine/article/0,9171,2011940,00.html. Accessed February 17, 2015.

2. Wax JR, Lucas FL, Lamont M, Pinette MG, Cartin A, Blackstone J. Maternal and newborn outcomes in planned home birth vs planned hospital births: a metaanalysis. *Am J Obstet Gynecol* 2010;203(3):243.e1–8.

3. A letter to *Time* on home birth. http://www.ourbodiesourselves.org/2010/10/a-letter-to-time-on-home-birth/. Accessed February 17, 2015.

4. UCLA Health website, Obstetrics and Gynecology page, Family Stories. http://obgyn.ucla.edu/body.cfm?id=174. Accessed February 15, 2014.

5. Fang YMV, Benn P, Campbell W, Bolnick J, Prabulos AM, Egan JFX. Down syndrome screening in the United States in 2001 and 2007: a survey of maternal-fetal medicine specialists. *Am J Obstet Gynecol* 2009;201(1):97.e1–5.

6. Midwives Alliance of North America. Statement of Values and Ethics. http://mana.org/pdfs/MANAStatementValuesEthicsColor.pdf. Accessed February 17, 2015.

7. Grossman D. *To the End of the Land*. New York, NY: Vintage, 2011:277.

Chapter 3

1. Ventura SJ, Mosher WD, Curtin SC, Abma JC, Henshaw S. Trends in pregnancies and pregnancy rates by outcome: Estimates for the United States, 1976–96. National Center for Health Statistics. Vital Health Stat 21(56); 2000.

2. Ventura SJ, Abma JC, Mosher WD, Henshaw SK. Estimated pregnancy rates for the United States, 1990–2005: An update. National vital statistics reports; vol 58 no 4. Hyattsville, MD: National Center for Health Statistics; 2009. http://www.cdc.gov/nchs/data/nvsr/nvsr58/nvsr58_04.pdf. Accessed February 17, 2015.

3. MacDorman MF, Kirmeyer S. Fetal and perinatal mortality, United States, 2005. National vital statistics reports; vol 57 no 8. Hyattsville, MD: National Center for Health Statistics; 2009.

4. Fretts RC, Schmittdiel J, McLean FH, Usher RH, Goldman MB. Increased maternal age and the risk of fetal death. *N Engl J Med* 1995;333:953–957.

5. Silver RM, Varner MW, Reddy U, et al. Work-up of stillbirth: a review of the evidence. *Am J Obstet Gynecol* 2007;196:433–444.

6. Brimacombe MB, Heller DS, Zamudio S. Comparison of fetal demise case series drawn from socioeconomically distinct counties in New Jersey. *Fetal Pediatr Pathol* 2007;26(5–6):213–222.

7. Varli IH, Petersson K, Bottinga R, et al. The Stockholm classification of stillbirth. *Acta Obstet Gynecol Scand* 2008;87:1202–1212.

8. Walsh CA, Vallerie AM, Baxi LV. Etiology of stillbirth at term: a 10-year cohort study. *J Matern Fetal Neonatal Med* 2008;21:493–501.

9. MacDorman MF, Munson ML, Kirmeyer S. Fetal and Perinatal Mortality, United States, 2004. National vital statistics reports; vol 56 no 3. Hyattsville, MD: National Center for Health Statistics; 2007.

10. Barfield W, Martin J, Hoyert D. Racial and ethnic trends in fetal mortality—United States, 1990–2000. *MMWR* 2004;53:529–530. http://www.cdc.gov/mmwr/pdf/wk/mm5324.pdf. Accessed February 17, 2015.

11. Fretts RC. Etiology and prevention of stillbirth. *Am J Obstet Gynecol* 2005;193:1923–1935.

Chapter 4

1. Kalish RB, Thaler HT, Chasen ST, et al. First- and second-trimester ultrasound assessment of gestational age. *Am J Obstet Gynecol* 2004;191:975–978.

2. Hoffman CS, Messer LC, Mendola P, Savitz DA, Herring AH, Hartmann KE. Comparison of gestational age at birth based on last menstrual period and ultrasound during the first trimester. *Paediatr Perinat Epidemiol* 2008;22:587–596.

3. Spong CY. Defining "term" pregnancy: recommendations from the Defining "Term" Pregnancy Workgroup. *JAMA* 2013;309:2445–2446.

4. Bird TM, Bronstein JM, Hall RW, Lowery CL, Nugent R, Mays GP. Late preterm infants: birth outcomes and health care utilization in the first year. *Pediatrics* 2010;126:e311-9.

5. Engle WA, Tomashek KM, Wallman C, and the Committee on the Fetus and Newborn. "Late-Preterm" infants: a population at risk. *Pediatrics* 2007;120:1390–1401.

6. Wang ML, Dorer DJ, Fleming MP, Catlin EA. Clinical outcomes of near-term infants. *Pediatrics* 2004;114:372–376.

7. Kramer MS, Demissie K, Yang H, et al. The contribution of mild and moderate preterm birth to infant mortality. Fetal and Infant Health Study Group of the Canadian Perinatal Surveillance System. *JAMA* 2000;284:843–849.

8. Hansen AK et al. Risk of respiratory morbidity in term infants delivered by elective caesarean section: cohort study. *BMJ* 2008;336:85–87.

9. Tita ATN, Landon MB, Spong CY, et al., for the Eunice Kennedy Shriver NICHD Maternal-Fetal Medicine Units Network. Timing of elective repeat cesarean delivery at term and neonatal outcomes. *N Engl J Med* 2009;360:111–120.

10. Engle WA. Infants born late preterm: definition, physiologic and metabolic immaturity, and outcomes. *NeoReviews* 2009;10:e280–286.

11. Wu JM, Hundley AF, Visco AG. Elective primary cesarean delivery: attitudes of urogynecology and maternal-fetal medicine specialists. *Obstet Gynecol* 2005;105(2):301–306.

Chapter 5

1. Centers for Disease Control and Prevention. Births—methods of delivery, 2012. CDC FastStats. http://www.cdc.gov/nchs/data/nvsr/nvsr62/nvsr62_09.pdf. Accessed February 17, 2015.

2. Centers for Disease Control and Prevention. Births—methods of delivery, 2011. CDC FastStats. http://www.cdc.gov/nchs/data/nvsr/nvsr62/nvsr62_01.pdf. Accessed February 17, 2015.

3. Declercq E, Menacker F, MacDorman MF. Rise in "no indicated risk" primary caesareans in the United States 1991–2001: cross sectional analysis. *BMJ* 2005;330:71–72.

4. Mason JO, McGinnis JM. "Healthy People 2000": an overview of the national health promotion and disease prevention objectives. *Public Health Rep* 1990;105(5):441–446.

5. U.S. Department of Health and Human Services. Healthy People 2010. Washington, DC: U.S. Department of Health and Human Services; 2000.

6. Kozhimannil KB, Law MR, Virnig BA. Cesarean delivery rates vary tenfold among U.S. hospitals; reducing variation may address quality and cost issues. *Health Affairs* 2013;32:527–535.

7. McPherson K, Strong PM, Epstein A, Jones L. Regional variations in the use of common surgical procedures: within and between England and Wales, Canada and the United States of America. *Soc Sci Med* 1981;15(3 Pt 1):273–288.

8. McKee M, Clarke E. Guidelines, enthusiasms, uncertainty, and the limits to purchasing. *BMJ* 1995;310:101–104.

9. Arrow, KJ. Uncertainty and the welfare economics of medical care. *Am Econ Rev* 1963;53: 941–973.

10. Gruber J, Woings M. Physician financial incentives and cesarean section delivery. *Rand J Econ* 1996:27:99–123.

11. Tussing AD, Wojtowycz MA. The cesarean decision in New York State, 1986. Economic and noneconomic aspects. *Med Care* 1992;30:529–540.

12. Tussing AD, Wojtowycz MA. Malpractice, defensive medicine, and obstetric behavior. *Med Care* 1997;35(2):172–191.

13. Benedetti TJ, Baldwin LM, Skillman SM, et al. Professional liability issues and practice patterns of obstetric providers in Washington State. *Obstet Gynecol* 2006;107:1238–1246.

14. Baldwin LM, Hart LG, Lloyd M, Fordyce M, Rosenblatt RA. Defensive medicine and obstetrics. *JAMA* 1995;274:1606–1610.

15. Entman SS, Glass CA, Hickson GB, Githens PB, Whetten-Goldstein K, Sloan FA. The relationship between malpractice claims history and subsequent obstetric care. *JAMA* 1994;272: 1588–1591.

16. Localio AR, Lawthers AG, Bengtson JM, et al. Relationship between malpractice claims and cesarean delivery. *JAMA* 1993;269:366–373.

17. Dubay L, Kaestner R, Waidmann T. The impact of malpractice fears on cesarean section rates. *J Health Econ* 1999;18:491–522.

18. Spetz J, Smith MW, Ennis MF. Physician incentives and the timing of cesarean sections: evidence from California. *Med Care* 2001;39:536–550.

19. Mayor S. Caesarean section rate in England reaches 22%. *BMJ* 2002;324(7346):1118.

20. Liu S, Rusen ID, Joseph KS, et al. Recent trends in caesarean delivery and indications for caesarean delivery in Canada. *J Obstet Gynaecol Can* 2004;26:735–742.

21. Villar J, Valladares E, Wojdyla D, et al., for the WHO 2005 global survey on maternal and perinatal health research group. Caesarean delivery rates and pregnancy outcomes: the 2005 WHO global survey on maternal and perinatal health in Latin America. Lancet 2006;367(9525):1819–1829.

22. Kosloske AM, Love CL, Rohrer JE, et al. The diagnosis of appendicitis in children: outcomes of a strategy based on pediatric surgical evaluation. *Pediatrics* 2004;113:29–34.

Chapter 6

1. Arms S. *Immaculate Deception: A New Look at Women and Childbirth in America*. Boston, MA: Houghton Mifflin; 1975.

2. Block J. *Pushed: The Painful Truth about Childbirth and Modern Maternity Care*. Philadelphia, PA: Da Capo Press; 2007:xxiv.

3. Martin E. *The Woman in the Body: A Cultural Analysis of Reproduction*. Boston, MA: Beacon Press, 1987:83.

4. Martin E. *The Woman in the Body: A Cultural Analysis of Reproduction*. Boston, MA: Beacon Press, 1987:83.

5. Martin E. Medical metaphors of women's bodies: menstruation and menopause. *Int J Health Serv* 1988;18:237–254.

6. Hyde A, Roche-Reid B. Midwifery practice and the crisis of modernity: implications for the role of the midwife. *Soc Sci Med* 2004;58:2613–2623.

7. Rothman BK. Women, providers, and control. *J Obstet Gynecol Neonatal Nursing* 1996; 25:253–256.

8. McCool WF, Simeone SA. Birth in the United States: an overview of trends past and present. *Nurs Clin N Am* 2002;43:250–261.

9. Mundy L. *Everything Conceivable: How Assisted Reproduction Is Changing Men, Women, and the World*. New York, NY: Knopf; 2007.

10. Mundy L. *Everything Conceivable: How Assisted Reproduction Is Changing Men, Women, and the World*. New York, NY: Knopf; 2007.

11. Markens S. *Surrogate Motherhood and the Politics of Reproduction*. Berkeley and Los Angeles: University of California Press; 2007.

12. Mitchell L. *Baby's First Picture: Ultrasound and the Politics of Fetal Subjects*. Toronto, ON: University of Toronto Press; 2001.

13. Franklin S, Roberts C. *Born and Made: An Ethnography of Preimplantation Genetic Diagnosis*. Princeton, NJ: Princeton University Press; 2006.

Chapter 7

1. American College of Obstetricians and Gynecologists. ACOG statement on Planned Home Birth. http://www.acog.org/Resources-And

-Publications/Committee-Opinions/Committee-on-Obstetric-Practice/
Planned-Home-Birth. Accessed February 17, 2015.

2. Cresswell JL, Stephens E. Home births. Joint Statement of the Royal
College of Obstetrics and Gynaecologists and Royal College of Midwives; 2007. https://www.rcm.org.uk/sites/default/files/home_births_
rcog_rcm0607.pdf. Accessed February 17, 2015.

3. Janssen PA, Saxell L, Page LA, Klein MC, Liston RM, Lee SK. Outcomes of planned home birth with registered midwife versus planned
hospital birth with midwife or physician. *CMAJ* 2009;181:377–383.

4. McLachlan H, Forster D. The safety of home birth: is the evidence
good enough? *CMAJ* 2009;181:359–360.

5. Lindgren HE, Radestad IJ, Christensson K, Hildingsson IM. Outcome
of planned home births compared to hospital births in Sweden between
1992 and 2004: a population-based register study. *Acta Obstet Gynecol
Scand* 2008;87:751–759.

6. Johnson KC, Daviss BA. Outcomes of planned home births with certified professional midwives: large prospective study in North America.
BMJ 2005;330(7505):1416.

7. Pang JW, Heffelfinger JD, Huang GJ, Benedetti TJ, Weiss NS. Outcomes of planned home births in Washington State: 1989–1996. *Obstet
Gynecol* 2002;100:253–259.

8. Olsen O, Clausen JA. Planned hospital birth versus planned home
birth. *Cochrane Database Syst Rev* 2012;9:CD000352. doi:10.1002/14651
858.CD000352.pub2.

9. De Vries R, Lemmens T. The social and cultural shaping of medical
evidence: case studies from pharmaceutical research and obstetric science. *Soc Sci Med* 2004;62:2694–2706.

10. De Vries R, Lemmens T. The social and cultural shaping of medical
evidence: case studies from pharmaceutical research and obstetric science. *Soc Sci Med* 2004;62:2694–2706.

11. VanWeel C, van der Velden K, Lagro-Janssen T. Home births revisited:
the continuing search for better evidence. *BJOG* 2009;116:1149–1150.

12. De Vries R. Midwifery in The Netherlands: vestige or vanguard? *Med Anthropol* 2001;20:277–311.

13. Mohangoo AD, Buitendijk SE, Hukkelhoven CW, et al. Higher perinatal mortality in The Netherlands than in other European countries: the Peristat-II study [article in Dutch]. *Ned Tijdschr Geneeskd* 2008;152:2718–2727.

14. Merkus JM. Obstetric care in The Netherlands under assessment again [article in Dutch]. *Ned Tijdschr Geneeskd* 2008;152(50):2707–2708.

Chapter 8

1. National Institutes of Health state-of-the-science conference statement: Cesarean delivery on maternal request March 27–29, 2006. *Obstet Gynecol* 2006;107:1386–1397.

2. Robson SJ, Tan WS, Adeyemi A, Dear KBG. Estimating the rate of cesarean section by maternal request: anonymous survey of obstetricians in Australia. *Birth* 2009;36:208–212.

3. Bettes BA, Coleman VH, Zinberg S, et al. Cesarean delivery on maternal request: obstetrician-gynecologists' knowledge, perception, and practice patterns. *Obstet Gynecol* 2007;109:57–66.

4. Tyagi V, Perera M, Guerrero K. Trends in obstretric anal sphincter injuries over 10 years. *J Obstet Gynaecol* 2013;33:844–849.

5. Memon HU, Handa VL. Vaginal childbirth and pelvic floor disorders. *Women's Health (London)* 2013;9:265–277.

6. Wu JM, Hundley AF, Visco AG. Elective primary cesarean delivery: attitudes of urogynecology and maternal-fetal medicine specialists. *Obstet Gynecol* 2005;105:301–306.

7. Hankins GD, Clark SM, Munn MB. Cesarean section on request at 39 weeks: impact on shoulder dystocia, fetal trauma, neonatal encephalopathy, and intrauterine fetal demise. *Semin Perinatol* 2006;30:276–287.

8. Copper RL, Goldenberg RL, DuBard MB, Davis RO. Risk factors for fetal death in white, black, and Hispanic women. Collaborative Group on Preterm Birth Prevention. *Obstet Gynecol* 1994;84:490–495.

9. Yudkin PL, Wood L, Redman CW. Risk of unexplained stillbirth at different gestational ages. *Lancet* 1987;1(8543):1192–1194.

Chapter 9

1. Landsteiner K, Wiener AS. An agglutination factor in human blood recognized by immune sera for rhesus blood. *P Soc Exp Biol Med* 1940;43:223–229.

2. Levine P, Stetson R. An unusual case of intra-group agglutination. *JAMA* 1939;113:126–127.

3. Bevis DCA. Composition of the liquor amnii in hemolytic disease of the newborn. *Lancet* 1950(September 30):443.

4. Liley AW. Intrauterine transfusion of the fetus in hemolytic disease. *BMJ* 1963(November 2): 1107.

5. Transfusion of a foetus. Editorial. *BMJ* 1963(November 2):1069.

6. Kunisaki SM, Jennings RW. Fetal surgery. *J Intensive Care Med* 2008;23:33–51.

7. Lejeune J, Gautier M, Turpin R. Les chromosomes humains en culture de tissue. *C R Hebd Seances Acad Sci* 1959;248:602–603.

8. Lejeune J, Gautier M, Turpin R. Étude des chromosomes somatiques de neuf enfants mongoliens. *C R Hebd Seances Acad Sci* 1959;248:1721–1722.

9. Gilgenkrantz S, Rivera EM. The history of cytogenetics. Portraits of some pioneers. *Ann Genet* 2003;46:433–442.

10. Jacobs PA, Baikie AG, Court Brown WM, Strong JA. The somatic chromosomes in mongolism. *Lancet* 1959;1(7075):710.

11. Steele MW, Breg WR. Chromosome analysis of human amniotic-fluid cells. *Lancet* 1966;287(7434):383–385.

12. Nadler HL. Antenatal detection of hereditary disorders. *Pediatrics* 1968;912–918.

13. Epstein CJ, Schneider EL, Conte FA, Friedman S. Prenatal detection of genetic disorders. *Am J Hum Genet* 1972;24:214–226.

14. The Three Missions of the Jerome Lejeune Foundation. http://www.fondationlejeune.org/en/our-missions-and-actions/care/the-three-missions-of-the-jerome-lejeune-institute Accessed February 17, 2015.

15. American Society of Human Genetics. The William Allan Award. http://www.ashg.org/pages/awards_overview.shtml.

16. Lejeune J. The William Allan Memorial Award Lecture. On the nature of men. *Am J Hum Genet* 1970;22:121–128.

17. National Association of Catholic Families. Professor Jerome Lejeune. http://www.cfnews.org.uk/lejeune.htm. Accessed September 18, 2010.

18. Gauthier M, Harper PS. Fiftieth anniversary of trisomy 21: returning to a discovery. *Hum Genet* 2009;126:317–324.

19. Dahm R. Friedrich Miescher and the discovery of DNA. *Dev Biol* 2005;278:274–288.

20. Maddox, B. The double helix and the 'wronged heroine.' *Nature* 2003;421:407.

21. Hook EB, Cross PK, Schreinemachers DM. Chromosomal abnormality rates at amniocentesis and in live-born infants. *JAMA* 1983;249:2034–2038.

Chapter 10

1. Junod SW, Marks L. Women's trials: the approval of the first oral contraceptive pill in the United States and Great Britain. *J Hist Med All Sci* 2002;57(2):117–160.

2. Watkins ES. *On the Pill: A Social History of Oral Contraceptives, 1950–1970*. Baltimore, MD: Johns Hopkins University Press; 1998:34.

3. Matthews TJ et al. Delayed childbearing. NCHS data brief no 21. Hyattsville, MD: National Center for Health Statistics; 2009.

4. The accident of birth. *Fortune* 1938(February):84.

5. Tone A. *Devices and Desires: A History of Contraceptives in America*. New York, NY: Hill and Wang; 2001:85.

6. Marks LV. *Sexual Chemistry: A History of the Contraceptive Pill*. New Haven and London: Yale University Press; 2001:52–53.

7. Pincus G. *The Control of Fertility*. New York, NY: Academic Press; 1965.

8. Djerassi C. *The Pill, Pygmy Chimps, and Degas' Horse*. New York, NY: Basic Books; 1998.

9. Rock J. *The Time Has Come: A Catholic Doctor's Proposal to End the Battle over Birth Control*. New York, NY: Knopf; 1963.

10. Tone A. *Devices and Desires: A History of Contraceptives in America*. New York, NY: Hill and Wang; 2001.

11. Watkins ES. *On the Pill: A Social History of Oral Contraceptives, 1950–1970*. Baltimore, MD: Johns Hopkins University Press; 1998.

12. PBS. *The Pill*. http://www.pbs.org/wgbh/amex/pill/filmmore/index.html. Accessed February 17, 2015 .

13. Marks LA. *Sexual Chemistry*. New Haven, CT: Yale University Press; 2001:116–137.

14. Watkins ES. *On the Pill: A Social History of Oral Contraceptives, 1950–1970*. Baltimore, MD: Johns Hopkins University Press; 1998.

15. NCBI. http://www.ncbi.nlm.nih.gov/pubmed?term=risk%20oral%20contraceptive. Accessed February 17, 2015 .

16. PBS. The Pill and the women's liberation movement. http://www.pbs.org/wgbh/amex/pill/peopleevents/e_lib.html. Accessed August 20, 2008.

17. Kantner JF, Zelnik M. Sexual and contraceptive experience of unmarried women in the United States, 1976 and 1971. *Fam Plann Perspect* 1977;9:55–71.

18. Barbato L. Study of the prescription and dispensing of contraceptive medications at institutions of higher education. *J Am Coll Health Assoc* 1971;19:303–306.

19. Hollis G, Lashman K. Family planning services in U.S. colleges and universities. *Fam Plann Perspect* 1974;6:173–175.

20. Goldin C, Katz L. The power of the pill: oral contraceptives and women's career and marriage decisions. *J Polit Econ* 2002;100:730–770.

21. Birdsall N, Chester LA. Contraception and the status of women: what is the link? *Fam Plann Perspect* 1987;19:14–18.

Chapter 11

1. Mather M. Fact Sheet: The decline in U.S. Fertility. World Population Data Sheet. Population Reference Bureau. http://www.prb.org/publications/datasheets/2012/world-population-data-sheet/fact-sheet-us-population.aspx. Accessed February 17, 2015.

2. D'Addio AC, D'Ercole MM. Trends and determinant of fertility rates in OECD countries: the role of policies. http://www.oecd.org/social/family/35304751.pdf; http://www.oecd.org/dataoecd/7/33/35304751.pdf. Accessed February 17, 2015 3. Heron M, Sutton PD, Xu J, Ventura, SJ, Strobino DM, Guyer B. Annual summary of vital statistics: 2007. *Pediatrics* 2010;125:4–15.

4. Guttmacher Institute. Induced abortion in the United States. http://www.guttmacher.org/pubs/fb_induced_abortion.html. Accessed February 15, 2014.

5. Ventura SJ, Abma JC, Mosher WD, Henshaw SK. Estimated pregnancy rates by outcome for the United States, 1990–2004. National vital statistics reports; vol 56 no 15. Hyattsville, MD: National Center for Health Statistics; 2008:1–25,28.

6. Livingston G, Cohn D. The new demography of American mother-hood. Washington, DC: Pew Research Center; 2010. http://www.pewsocialtrends.org/2010/05/06/the-new-demography-of-american-motherhood/. Accessed February 15, 2014.

7. Livingston G, Cohn D. U.S. birth rate falls to a record low; decline is greatest among immigrant women. Washington, DC: Pew Research Center; 2012. http://www.pewsocialtrends.org/2012/11/29/u-s-birth-rate-falls-to-a-record-low-decline-is-greatest-among-immigrants/. Accessed July 7, 2014.

8. Matthews TJ et al. Delayed childbearing. NCHS data brief no 21. Hyattsville, MD: National Center for Health Statistics; 2009. http://www.cdc.gov/nchs/data/databriefs/db21.pdf. Accessed March 12, 2014.

9. Martin JA, Hamilton BE, Osterman MJK, Curtin SC, Mathews TJ. Births: Final data for 2012. National vital statistics reports; vol 62 no 9. Hyattsville, MD: National Center for Health Statistics; 2013. http://www.cdc.gov/nchs/data/nvsr/nvsr62/nvsr62_09.pdf. Accessed July 7, 2014.

10. Ventura SJ, Abma JC, Mosher WD, Henshaw SK. Estimated pregnancy rates by outcome for the United States, 1990–2004. National vital statistics reports; vol 56 no 15. Hyattsville MD: National Center for Health Statistics; 2008.

11. Ventura SJ. Changing Patterns of Nonmarital Childbearing in the United States. NCHS data brief no 18. Hyattsville, MD: National Center for Health Statistics; 2009.

12. Minnesota Legislative Commission on the Economic Status of Women. Fertility and birth rates in the U.S. and MN. MLCESW newsletter no 256; 2001. http://www.commissions.leg.state.mn.us/oesw/newsletters_/dec01.pdf. Accessed December 6, 2010.

13. Heron M, Sutton PD, Xu J, Ventura SJ, Strobino DM, Guyer B. Annual summary of vital statistics: 2007. *Pediatrics* 2010;125:4–15.

Chapter 12

1. Cnattingius S, Forman MR, Berendes HW, Isotalo L. Delayed child-bearing and risk of adverse perinatal outcome: a population-based study. *JAMA* 1992;268:886–890.

2. Astolfi P, De Pasquale A, Zonta L. Late childbearing and its impact on adverse pregnancy outcome: stillbirth, preterm delivery and low birth weight. *Rev Epidemiol Sante* 2005;53(Spec no 2):2S97–105.

3. Aldous MB, Edmonson MB. Maternal age at first childbirth and risk of low birth weight and preterm delivery in Washington State. *JAMA* 1993;270:2574–2577.

4. Tough SC, Newburn-Cook C, Johnston DW, Svenson LW, Rose S, Belik J. Delayed childbearing and its impact on population rate changes in lower birth weight, multiple birth, and preterm delivery. *Pediatrics* 2002;109:399–403.

5. Huang L, Sauve R, Birkett N, Fergusson D, van Walraven C. Maternal age and risk of stillbirth: a systematic review. *CMAJ* 2008;178:165–172.

6. Joseph KS, Allen AC, Dodds L, Turner LA, Scott H, Liston R. The perinatal effects of delayed childbearing. *Obstet Gynecol* 2006;105:1410–1418.

7. Tough SC, Newburn-Cook C, Johnston DW, Svenson LW, Rose S, Belik J. Delayed childbearing and its impact on population rate changes in lower birth weight, multiple birth, and preterm delivery. *Pediatrics* 2002;109:399–403.

8. Newburn-Cook CV, Onyskiw JE. Is older maternal age a risk factor for preterm birth and fetal growth restriction? A systematic review. *Health Care Women Int* 2005;26:852–875.

Chapter 13

1. Johnson JA, Tough S; Society of Obstetricians and Gynaecologists of Canada. Delayed child-bearing. *J Obstet Gynaecol Can* 2012;34:80–93.

2. McDonald JW, Rosina A, Rizzi E, Colombo B. Age and fertility: can women wait until their early thirties to try for a first birth? *J Biosoc Sci* 2011;43:685–700.

3. Abma J, Chandra A, Mosher W, Peterson L, Piccinino L. Fertility, family planning, and women's health: New data from the 1995 National Survey of Family Growth. National Center for Health Statistics. Vital Health Stat 23(19); 1997.

4. Lisonkova S, Joseph KS. Temporal trends in clomiphene citrate use: a population-based study. *Fertil Steril* 2012;97:639–644.

5. Wang H, Land JA, Bos HJ, Bakker MK, de Jong-van den Berg LT. Clomiphene citrate utilization in the Netherlands 1998–2007. *Hum Reprod.* 2011;26:1227–1231.

6. Centers for Disease Control and Prevention. Assisted reproductive technology. http://www.cdc.gov/art/ART2010/section1.htm. Accessed February 15, 2014.

7. Schieve LA, Devine O, Boyle CA, Petrini JR, Warner L. Estimation of the contribution of non-assisted reproductive technology ovulation stimulation fertility treatments to U.S. singleton and multiple births. *Am J Epidemiol* 2009;170:1396–1407.

8. Kulkarni AD, Jamieson DJ, Jones HW Jr, Kissin DM, Gallo MF, Macaluso M, Adashi EY. Fertility treatments and multiple births in the United States. *N Engl J Med* 2013;369:2218–2225.

9. Martin JA, Hamilton BE, Osterman MJK. Three decades of twin births in the United States, 1980–2009. NCHS data brief no 80. Hyattsville, MD: National Center for Health Statistics; 2012.

10. Sunderam S, Chang J, Flowers L, et al. Assisted reproductive technology surveillance—United States, 2006. *MMWR Surveill Summ* 2009;58:1–25.

Chapter 14

1. Joseph KS, Kramer MS, Marcoux S, Ohlsson A, Wen SW, Allen A, Platt R. Determinants of preterm birth rates in Canada from 1981 through 1983 and from 1992 through 1994. *N Engl J Med* 1998;339:1434–1439.

2. Blondel B, Kogan MD, Alexander GR, et al. The impact of the increasing number of multiple births on the rates of preterm birth and low birthweight: an international study. *Am J Public Health* 2002;92:1323–1330.

3. VanderWeele TJ, Lantos JD, Lauderdale DS. Rising preterm birth rates, 1989–2004: changing demographics or changing obstetric practice? *Soc Sci Med* 2012;74(2):196–201.

4. MacDorman MF, Declercq E, Zhang J. Obstetrical intervention and the singleton preterm birth rate in the United States from 1991 to 2006. *Am J Public Health* 2010;100:2241–2247.

5. Ananth CV, Joseph KS, Oyelese Y, Demissie K, Vintzileos A. Trends in preterm birth and perinatal mortality among singletons: United States, 1989 through 2000. *Obstet Gynecol* 2005;105:1084–1091.

Chapter 15

1. American College of Obstetricians and Gynecologists Committee on Practice Bulletins. ACOG Practice Bulletin No. 107: Induction of labor. *Obstet Gynecol* 2009;114(2 Pt 1):386.

Chapter 16

1. Sachs BP, Layde PM, Rubin GL, Rochat RW. Reproductive mortality in the United States. *JAMA* 1982;247:2789–2792.

2. Joseph KS. Theory of obstetrics: an epidemiologic framework for justifying medically indicated early delivery. *BMC Pregnancy Childbirth* 2007;7:4–19.

3. Joseph KS, Liu S, Rouleau J, et al.; Fetal and Infant Health Study Group of the Canadian Perinatal Surveillance System. Influence of definition based versus pragmatic birth registration on international comparisons of perinatal and infant mortality: population based retrospective study. *BMJ* 2012;344:e746. doi:10.1136/bmj.e746.

Chapter 17

1. Anderson EW, Ibsen B. The anesthetic management of patients with poliomyelitis and respiratory paralysis. *BMJ* 1954; 1(4865):786–788.

2. Snider GL. Historical perspective on mechanical ventilation: from simple life support system to ethical dilemma. *Am Rev Respir Dis.* 1989;140(2 Pt 2):S2–7.

3. Singh GK, van Dyck PC. *Infant Mortality in the United States, 1935–2007: Over Seven Decades of Progress and Disparities.* Rockville, MD: U.S. Department of Health and Human Services; 2010. http://www.hrsa.gov/ healthit/images/mchb_infantmortality_pub.pdf. Accessed July 29, 2013.

4. Korst LM, Fridman M, Lu MC, Fleege L, Mitchell C, Gregory KD. Trending elective preterm deliveries using administrative data. *Paediatr Perinat Epidemiol* 2013;27:44–53.

Chapter 18

1. West M. *Prenatal Care.* Washington, DC: U.S. Dept of Labor Children's Bureau; 1913. http://mchlibrary.info/history/chbu/2265-1913. PDF. Accessed November 23, 2012.

2. West M. *Prenatal Care.* Washington, DC: U.S. Dept of Labor Children's Bureau; 1913:12. http://mchlibrary.info/history/chbu/2265-1913. PDF. Accessed November 23, 2012.

3. Prenatal care fact sheet. http://womenshealth.gov/publications/our -publications/fact-sheet/prenatal-care.cfm. Accessed February 17, 2015.

4. Consensus conference: the use of diagnostic ultrasound imaging during pregnancy. *JAMA* 1984;252:669–672.

5. Ewigman BG, Crane JP, Frigoletto FD, LeFevre ML, Bain RP, McNellis D. Effect of prenatal ultrasound screening on perinatal outcome. RADIUS Study Group. *N Engl J Med* 1993;329:821–827.

6. Grandjean H, Larroque D, Levi S. The performance of routine ultrasonographic screening of pregnancies in the Eurofetus Study. *Am J Obstet Gynecol* 1999;181:446–454.

7. Woodward RS. Controlling health expenditures. *N Engl J Med* 2001;345:770–772.

8. Siddique J, Lauderdale DS, VanderWeele TJ, Lantos JD. Trends in prenatal ultrasound use in the United States: 1995 to 2006. *Med Care* 2009;47:1129–1135.

9. Colby CE, Carey WA, Blumenfeld YJ, Hintz SR. Infants with prenatally diagnosed anomalies: special approaches to preparation and resuscitation. *Clin Perinatol* 2012;39:871–877.

10. Sutton LN, Adzick NS, Bilaniuk LT, Johnson MP, Crombleholme TM, Flake AW. Improvement in hindbrain herniation demonstrated by serial fetal magnetic resonance imaging following fetal surgery for myelomeningocele. *JAMA* 1999;282(19):1826–1831.

11. Bruner JP, Tulipan N, Paschall RL, et al. Fetal surgery for myelomeningocele and the incidence of shunt-dependent hydrocephalus. *JAMA* 1999;282(19):1819–1825.

12. Johnson CY, Honein MA, Dana Flanders W, Howards PP, Oakley GP Jr, Rasmussen SA. Pregnancy termination following prenatal diagnosis of anencephaly or spina bifida: a systematic review of the literature. *Birth Defects Res A Clin Mol Teratol* 2012;94:857–863.

13. Davis BE, Daley CM, Shurtleff DB, et al. Long-term survival of individuals with myelomeningocele. *Pediatr Neurosurg* 2005;41(4):186–191. doi:10.1159/000086559.

14. Smithells RW, Sheppard S, Schorah CJ, et al. Possible prevention of neural-tube defects by periconceptional vitamin supplementation. *Lancet* 1980;1(8164):339–340. doi:10.1016/S0140-6736(80)90886-7.

15. Dias MS. Neurosurgical management of myelomeningocele (spina bifida). *Pediatr Rev* 2005;26(2):50–60. doi:10.1542/pir.26-2-50.

16. Morris JK, Wald NJ. Quantifying the decline in the birth prevalence of neural tube defects in England and Wales. *J Med Screen.* 1999;6:182–185.

17. Macri JN, Weiss RR. Prenatal serum alpha-fetoprotein screening for neural tube defects. *Obstet Gynecol* 1982;59:633–639.

18. Holtzman NA, Leonard CO, Farfel MR. Issues in antenatal and neonatal screening and surveillance for hereditary and congenital disorders. *Annu Rev Publ Health* 1981;2:219–251. doi:10.1146/annurev.pu.02.050181.001251.

19. Brock DJ, Scrimgeour JB, Steven J, Barron L, Watt M. Maternal plasma alpha-fetoprotein screening for fetal neural tube defects. *BJOG* 1978;85:575–581.

20. Campbell S, Pryse-Davies J, Coltart TM, Seller MJ, Singer JD. Ultrasound in diagnosis of spina bifida. *Lancet* 1975;305(7915):1065–1068.

21. Cameron M, Martin P. Prenatal screening and diagnosis of neural tube defects. *Prenatal Diag* 2009;29:402–411.

22. Sutton LN, Adzick NS, Bilaniuk LT, Johnson MP, Crombleholme TM, Flake AW. Improvement in hindbrain herniation demonstrated by serial fetal magnetic resonance imaging following fetal surgery for myelomeningocele. *JAMA* 1999;282:1826–1831.

23. Meuli M, Moehrlen U. Fetal surgery for myelomeningocele: a critical appraisal. *Eur J Pediatr Surg* 2013;23:103–109.

24. Bruner JP, Tulipan N, Paschall RL, et al. Fetal surgery for myelomeningocele and the incidence of shunt-dependent hydrocephalus. *JAMA* 1999;282(19):1819–1825. doi:10.1001/jama.282.19.1819.

25. Johnson MP, Sutton LN, Rintoul N, et al. Fetal myelomeningocele repair: short-term clinical outcomes. *Am J Obstet Gynecol* 2003;189(2):482–487.

26. Adzick NS, Thom EA, Spong CY, et al. A randomized trial of prenatal versus postnatal repair of myelomeningocele. *N Engl J Med* 2011;364(11):993–1004.

27. Meuli M, Moehrlen U. Fetal surgery for myelomeningocele: a critical appraisal. *Eur J Pediatr Surg* 2013;23(2):103–109. doi:10.1055/s-0033-1343082.

28. Johnson MP, Sutton LN, Rintoul N, et al. Fetal myelomeningocele repair: short-term clinical outcomes. *Am J Obstet Gynecol* 2003;189(2):482–487.

29. Sutton LN, Adzick NS, Bilaniuk LT, Johnson MP, Crombleholme TM, Flake AW. Improvement in hindbrain herniation demonstrated by serial fetal magnetic resonance imaging following fetal surgery for myelomeningocele. *JAMA* 1999;282(19):1826–1831. doi:10.1001/jama.282.19.1826.

30. Adzick, NS. Fetal surgery for spina bifida: past, present, future. *Semin Pediatr Surg* 2013;22(1):10–17.

31. Brezinka, C. Reading the EUROCAT study. *Ultrasound Obst Gyn* 2005;25:3–5.

32. Wilson MS, Carroll MA, Braun SA, et al. Is preterm delivery indicated in fetuses with gastroschisis and antenatally detected bowel dilation? *Fetal Diagn Ther* 2012;32:262–266.

33. Hon EH. Apparatus for continuous monitoring of the fetal heart rate. *Yale J Biol Med* 1960;32:397–399.

34. Hon EH, Hess OW. The clinical value of fetal electrocardiography. *Am J Obstet Gynecol* 1960;79:1012–1023.

35. Lee WK, Baggish MS. The effect of unselected intrapartum fetal monitoring. *Obstet Gynecol* 1976;47(5):516–520.

36. McCusker J, Harris DR, Hosmer DW Jr. Association of electronic fetal monitoring during labor with cesaren section rate and with neonatal morbidity and mortality. *Am J Public Health* 1988;78:1170–1174.

37. Alfirevic Z, Devane D, Gyte GM. Continuous cardiotocography (CTG) as a form of electronic fetal monitoring (EFM) for fetal assessment during labor. *Cochrane Database Syst Rev* 2013;5:CD006066. doi:10.1002/14651858.CD006066.pub2.

38. Siddique J, Lauderdale DS, VanderWeele TJ, Lantos JD. Trends in prenatal ultrasound use in the United States: 1995 to 2006. *Med Care* 2009;47:1129–1135.

39. Chen HY, Chauhan SP, Ananth CV, Vintzileos AM, Abuhamad AZ. Electronic fetal heart rate monitoring and its relationship to neonatal and infant mortality in the United States. *Am J Obstet Gynecol* 2011;204(6):491.e1–10.

40. Devoe LD. Electronic fetal monitoring: does it really lead to better outcomes? *Am J Obstet Gynecol* 201;204:455–456.

Chapter 19

1. Heisler EJ. The U.S. Infant mortality rate: International comparisons, underlying factors, and federal programs. Congressional Research Service; 2012. http://www.fas.org/sgp/crs/misc/R41378.pdf. Accessed August 2, 2013.

2. MacDorman MF, Mathews TJ. Behind international rankings of infant mortality: How the United States compares with Europe. NCHS data brief no 23. Hyattsville, MD: National Center for Health Statistics; 2009.

3. Dolk H, Loane M, Garne E. The prevalence of congenital anomalies in Europe. *Adv Exp Med Biol* 2010;686:349–364.

4. Leroi, AM. The future of neo-eugenics. *EMBO Rep* 2006 Dec; 7(12): 1184–1187.

Chapter 20

1. Dubay L, Joyce T, Kaestner R, Kenney GM. Changes in prenatal care timing and low birth weight by race and socioeconomic status: implications for the Medicaid expansions for pregnant women. *Health Serv Res* 2001;36:373–398.

2. Ray WA, Mitchel EF Jr, Piper JM. Effect of Medicaid expansions on preterm birth. *Am J Prev Med.* 1997;13(4):292–297.

3. Kaestner R. Health insurance, the quantity and quality of prenatal care, and infant health. *Inquiry* 1999;36:162–175.

4. Vintzileos A, Ananth CV, Smulian JC, Scorza WE, Knuppel RA. The impact of prenatal care on postneonatal deaths in the presence and absence of antenatal high-risk conditions. *Am J Obstet Gynecol* 2002;187:1258–1262.

5. Stevens-Simon C. Low-birthweight prevention programs: the enigma of failure. *Birth* 1999;26:184–191.

6. Lu MC, Tache V, Alexander GR, Kotelchuck M, Halfon N. Preventing low birth weight: is prenatal care the answer? *J Matern Fetal Neonatal Med* 2003;13:362–380.

7. Huntington J, Connell F. For every dollar spent: the cost-savings argument for prenatal care. *N Engl J Med* 1994;331:1303–1307.

8. Kochanek KD, Martin JA. Supplemental analyses of recent trends in infant mortality. National Center for Health Statistics; 2004. http://www.cdc.gov/nchs/data/hestat/infantmort/infantmort.htm.

9. Hoyert DL, Xu J. Deaths: Preliminary data for 2011. National vital statistics reports; vol 61 no 6. Hyattsville, MD: National Center for Health Statistics; 2012.

10. CDC Grand Rounds: public health approaches to reducing U.S. infant mortality. *MMWR* 2013;62(31);625–628.

11. Martin JA, Hamilton BE, Osterman MJK, Curtin SC, Mathews TJ. Births: Final data for 2012. National vital statistics reports; vol 62 no 9. Hyattsville, MD: National Center for Health Statistics; 2013.

12. Been JV, Nurmatov UB, Cox B, et al. Effect of smoke-free legislation on perinatal and child health: a systematic review and meta-analysis. *Lancet* 2014;383(9928):1549–1560.

Index

Basic Bioethics
Arthur Caplan, editor

Books Acquired under the Editorship of Glenn McGee and Arthur Caplan

Peter A. Ubel, *Pricing Life: Why It's Time for Health Care Rationing*

Mark G. Kuczewski and Ronald Polansky, eds., *Bioethics: Ancient Themes in Contemporary Issues*

Suzanne Holland, Karen Lebacqz, and Laurie Zoloth, eds., *The Human Embryonic Stem Cell Debate: Science, Ethics, and Public Policy*

Gita Sen, Asha George, and Piroska Östlin, eds., *Engendering International Health: The Challenge of Equity*

Carolyn McLeod, *Self-Trust and Reproductive Autonomy*

Lenny Moss, *What Genes Can't Do*

Jonathan D. Moreno, ed., *In the Wake of Terror: Medicine and Morality in a Time of Crisis*

Glenn McGee, ed., *Pragmatic Bioethics, second edition*

Timothy F. Murphy, *Case Studies in Biomedical Research Ethics*

Mark A. Rothstein, ed., *Genetics and Life Insurance: Medical Underwriting and Social Policy*

Kenneth A. Richman, *Ethics and the Metaphysics of Medicine: Reflections on Health and Beneficence*

David Lazer, ed., *DNA and the Criminal Justice System: The Technology of Justice*

Harold W. Baillie and Timothy K. Casey, eds., *Is Human Nature Obsolete? Genetics, Bioengineering, and the Future of the Human Condition*

Books Acquired under the Editorship of Arthur Caplan

Timothy F. Murphy, *Ethics, Sexual Orientation, and Choices about Children*

Daniel Callahan, *In Search of the Good: A Life in Bioethics*

Robert Blank, *Intervention in the Brain: Politics, Policy, and Ethics*

Gregory E. Kaebnick and Thomas H. Murray, eds., *Synthetic Biology and Morality: Artificial Life and the Bounds of Nature*

Dominic A. Sisti, Arthur L. Caplan, and Hila Rimon-Greenspan, eds., *Applied Ethics in Mental Health Care: An Interdisciplinary Reader*

Barbara K. Redman, *Research Misconduct Policy in Biomedicine: Beyond the Bad-Apple Approach*

Russell Blackford, *Humanity Enhanced: Genetic Choice and the Challenge for Liberal Democracies*

Nicholas Agar, *Truly Human Enhancement: A Philosophical Defense of Limits*

Bruno Perreau, *The Politics of Adoption: Gender and the Making of French Citizenship*

Carl E. Schneider, *The Censor's Hand: The Misregulation of Human-Subject Research*

Lydia Dugdale, ed., *Dying in the Twenty-First Century: Toward a New Ethical Framework for the Art of Dying Well*

John D. Lantos and Diane S. Lauderdale, *Preterm Babies, Fetal Patients, and Childbearing Choices*

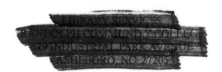
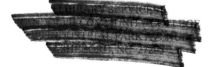